Teaching Atlas
of Mammography

Fortschritte auf dem Gebiete der Röntgenstrahlen und der Nuklearmedizin

Diagnostik, Physik, Biologie, Therapie

Supplement
Volume 116

Edited by
W. Frommhold
and P. Thurn

In Collaboration with
G. Breitling, E. Vogler
and K. zum Winkel

1985
Georg Thieme Verlag
Stuttgart · New York

Thieme Inc.
New York

Teaching Atlas of Mammography

By László Tabár and
Peter B. Dean

2nd revised edition
419 partly colored figures

1985
Georg Thieme Verlag
Stuttgart · New York

Thieme Inc.
New York

Docent László Tabár, M. D.

Department of Mammography
Falun Central Hospital
S-79 182 Falun, Sweden

Docent Peter B. Dean, M. D.

Department of Diagnostic Radiology
University Central Hospital
SF-20 520 Turku 52, Finland

CIP-Kurztitelaufnahme der Deutschen Bibliothek

Tabár, László:
Teaching atlas of mammography / by László Tabár and
Peter B. Dean. − 2. rev. ed. − Stuttgart ; New York :
Thieme ; New York : Thieme-Stratton, 1985.
  (Fortschritte auf dem Gebiete der Röntgenstrahlen
  und der Nuklearmedizin : Supplement ; Vol. 116)
NE: Dean, Peter B.:; Fortschritte auf dem Gebiete der
Röntgenstrahlen und der Nuklearmedizin / Ergänzungs-
band

Important Note:

Medicine is an ever-changing science. Research and clinical experience are continually broadening our knowledge, in particular our knowledge of proper treatment and drug therapy. Insofar as this book mentions any dosage or application, readers may rest assured that the authors, editors and publishers have made every effort to ensure that such references are strictly in accordance with the state of knowledge at the time of production of the book. Nevertheless, every user is requested to carefully examine the manufacturers' leaflets accompanying each drug to check on his own responsibility whether the dosage schedules recommended therein of the contraindications stated by the manufacturers differ from the statements made in the present book. Such examination is particularly important with drugs which are either rarely used or have been newly released on the market.

1st edition 1983   1st German edition 1985

© 1983, 1985 Georg Thieme Verlag, Rüdigerstr. 14, D-7000 Stuttgart 30
Printed in Germany

Typesetting by Maschinensetzerei Hurler, D-7311 Notzingen (Linotron 202).
Printing by Karl Grammlich, D-7401 Pliezhausen.

ISBN 3-13-640802-0   Georg Thieme Verlag   ISBN 0-86577-198-7   Thieme Inc., New York
ISSN 0342-6114   Stuttgart · New York   LC 83-050659

6 5 4

This book is dedicated to
Viktória and Arja

Preface to the Second Edition

This atlas consists of a systematic collection of mammograms of breast lesions, many in the early and some in the earliest detectable phases of development. These reflect the types of lesions to be found in a mammography screening population. Small malignant lesions are presumed to be the precursors of large, metastasizing lesions, and their removal at a sufficiently early stage should prevent the development of breast cancer to the stage where it kills the patient.

There is no question that mammography screening, when performed to high standards and repeated at sufficiently frequent intervals, leads to the detection of most breast cancers at a preclinical stage. The result is a lower mortality from breast cancer and, in many cases, less mutilating and traumatic therapy than previously possible.

This book was written to help radiologists fill the anticipated need for many skilled mammographers. We expect that this need will continue to grow as population screening with mammography becomes more widely adopted. This edition contains no major revisions and no additional figures. We are grateful to many of our colleagues for constructive criticism, and with the publication of this second edition we have endeavoured to respond to their comments.

Falun, Sweden
Turku, Finland
February 1986

László Tabár
Peter B. Dean

Introduction

The purpose of this Atlas is to teach radiologists how to analyze mammograms and arrive at the correct diagnosis through proper evaluation of the findings. The illustrated cases cover practically the entire spectrum of breast abnormalities. They are based upon referred patient material as well as 80,000 mammographic screening examinations.

There are two basic steps in the interpretation of mammograms: perception and analysis.

Since the greatest benefit of mammography lies in the detection of breast carcinoma in its earliest possible stages, every mammogram must be systematically surveyed for the subtle hints of malignancy. Perception is taught in this Atlas by describing a method for systematic viewing (Chapter 2). The reader is then provided with a series of mammograms with obscure lesions to encourage practice with this method. With the help of a coordinate system, the lesions can be precisely located. Practice in perception continues throughout the Atlas. After detecting an abnormality on the mammogram, the diagnosis can be reached through a careful analysis of the X-ray signs. Additional projections, coned-down compression and magnification views provide further help in this analytic workup.

Rather than starting with the diagnosis and demonstrating typical findings, the approach of this Atlas is to teach the reader how to analyze the image and reach the correct diagnosis through proper evaluation of the X-ray signs. Prerequisites for the perception and evaluation of the X-ray signs are optimum technique, knowledge of anatomy and understanding of the pathological processes leading to the mammographic appearances.

Contents

I. Anatomy of the Breast 1
II. Method for Systematic Viewing of Mammograms 5
III. Approach to Mammographic Film Interpretation 15
IV. Circumscribed Lesions 17
    Signs of Primary Importance in Diagnosing Circumscribed Tumors 18
    Signs of Secondary Importance in Diagnosing Circumscribed Lesions . . 19
    Practice in Analyzing Circumscribed Tumors (Cases 1–56) 21
V. Stellate Lesions 87
    Key Case 91
    Practice in Analyzing Stellate Lesions (Cases 58–85) 92
VI. Calcifications 137
    Ductal-type Calcifications 138
Practice in Calcification Analysis (Cases 86–109) 140
Lobular Type Calcifications 170
Miscellaneous Calcifications 172
Practice in Calcification Analysis (Cases 112–152) 174
VII. Thickened Skin Syndrome of the Breast 211
VIII. Overall Strategy 217

References 219
Index 221

Color Plates I and II after Page 136

I. Anatomy of the Breast

This description is based upon the recent work of Wellings (48, 49, 50) and Azzopardi (4) who have done much to clarify the anatomic structure of the breast.

Anatomically the breast can be subdivided into the following structural entities:

Lobe (Fig. I): The human breast contains 15–18 lobes. Each lobe has a main duct opening in the nipple.

Terminal ductal lobular unit (TDLU) (Fig. II): The main duct branches and eventually forms the terminal ductal lobular unit (TDLU), consisting of the extralobular terminal duct and the lobule (48).

Lobule: The intralobular terminal duct and ductules surrounded by a special, loose intralobular connective tissue form a lobule (Fig. II). In some nomenclature the ductules correspond to acini (4).

The extralobular and intralobular terminal ducts can be identified by two characteristics:

— The extralobular terminal duct is surrounded by elastic tissue while the intralobular terminal duct and ductules are not.

— The extralobular terminal duct is lined by columnar cells while the intralobular terminal duct contains cuboidal cells (4).

The anatomic details are important since certain breast diseases arise from specific anatomic locations (4, 50):

Main duct and its branches:

a) Benign papilloma and malignant papillary tumors arise preferentially in the larger ducts.

b) duct ectasia is primarily a disease of the ducts. Dilitation

Terminal ductal lobular unit (TDLU): According to Wellings (50), the terminal ductal lobular unit is of central importance because it is the site of origin of:

a) Ductal carcinoma in situ,

b) lobular carcinoma in situ,

c) infiltrating ductal carcinoma,

d) infiltrating lobular carcinoma,

e) fibroadenoma,

f) most components of fibrocystic disease (cysts, apocrine metaplasia, various forms of adenosis, epitheliosis).

"It is our belief that the epithelial hyperplasias that are precancerous arise in the TDLU, within the lobular portion or in the terminal duct or both. Larger ducts can be ruled out as common origins of precancer and cancer." (50) "Intraductal proliferative lesions most commonly affect the terminal ducts at the point where the elastic mantle surrounding the duct disappears and the duct joins the lobule". (10)

g) Cysts originate in the lobules; their size may range up to several centimeters. Apocrine transformation of the lobular epithelium results in increased fluid secretion. Blockage of the extralobular terminal duct by external fibrosis or internal processes (intraductal epithelial proliferation) leads to dilatation of the lobule into a tension cyst (4) (Fig. III).

Explanation of terms:

Adenosis (Fig. IV): The glandular structures proliferate, resulting in the production of new ductules and lobules.

Epitheliosis: The epithelial cells proliferate within preexisting ducts and lobules.

Cystic hyperplasia (Fibrocystic disease) (Fig. V A, V B): Includes epithelial cysts, fibrosis, apocrine metaplasia, various forms of adenosis and epitheliosis.

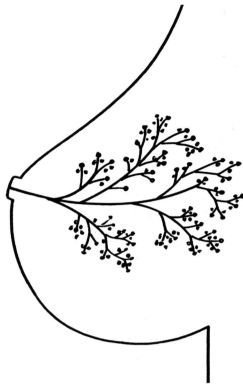

Fig. I: Diagram of the breast illustrating a single lobe.

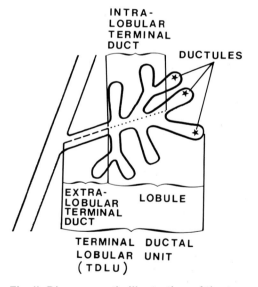

Fig. II: Diagrammatic illustration of the terminal ductal lobular unit (adapted from Wellings).

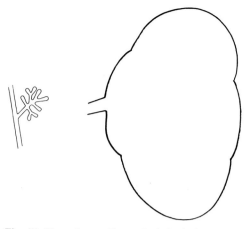

Fig. III: Transformation of a lobule into a
tension cyst.

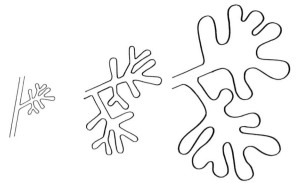

Fig. IV: Development of adenosis.

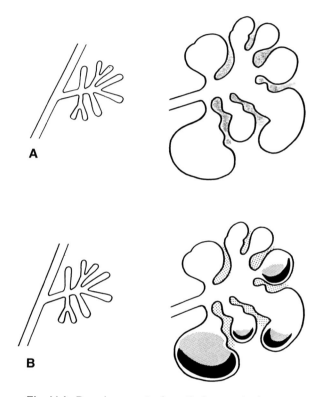

A

B

Fig. V A: Development of cystic hyperplasia.

Fig. V B: Development of cystic hyperplasia with
calcifications.

II. Method for Systematic Viewing of Mammograms

A detailed comparison of the left and right breasts enhances the detection of structural asymmetries. Perception of subtle alterations can be accentuated by sequential viewing of restricted areas of the mammograms, as follows.

Masking:
a) Horizontal masking: caudal (Fig. VI) and cranial (Fig. VII) aspects,
b) oblique masking: cranial (Fig. VIII) and caudal (Fig. IX) aspects.

Searching for **asymmetric densities** within the parenchyma (Fig. X).

Comparison of parenchymal **contours:**
a) Local retraction of the parenchymal contour on the cranio-caudal projection (Fig. XI),
b) local retraction of the parenchymal contour on the medio-lateral or latero-medial projections (Fig. XII).

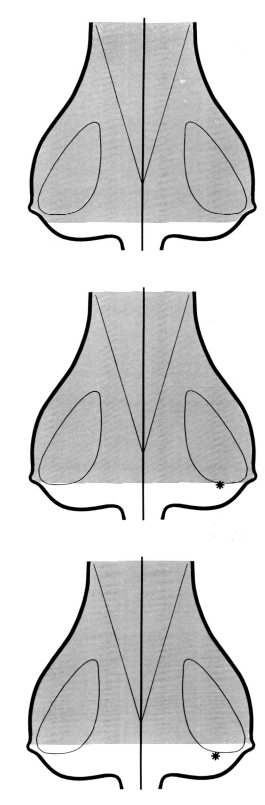

Fig. VI: Horizontal masking, caudal aspect. Stepwise horizontal masking facilitates the comparison of corresponding regions of the two breasts. The shaded region is covered by an opaque sheet of cardboard, paper, or film, which is gradually moved in the cranial direction to expose the caudal border of the breast.

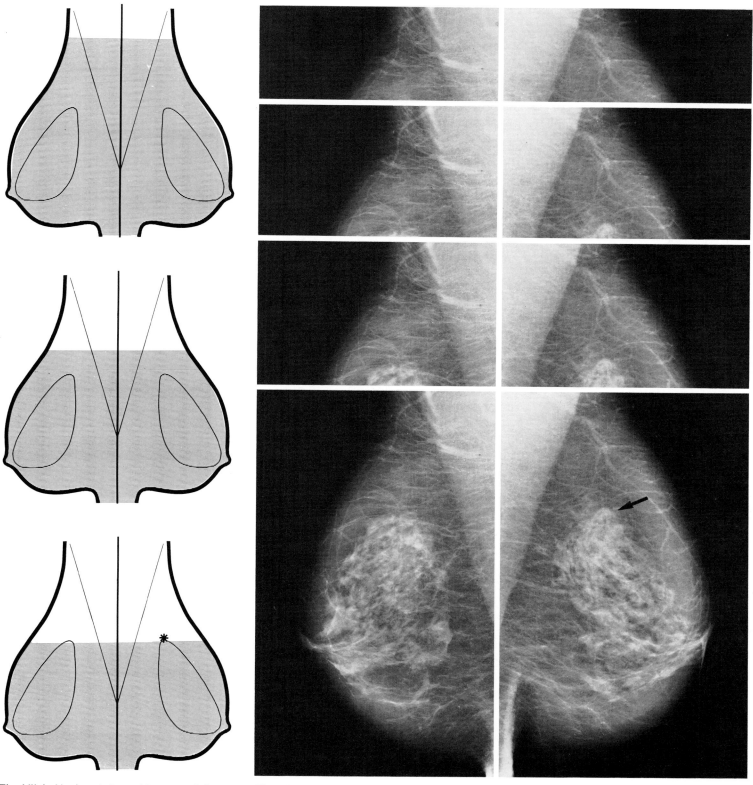

Fig. VII A: Horizontal masking, cranial aspect. Right and left mammograms of the medio-lateral oblique (or latero-medial) projections are viewed. Stepwise horizontal masking facilitates the comparison of corresponding regions of the two breasts.

Fig. VII B: Horizontal masking, cranial aspect, demonstrated on the medio-lateral oblique views of case 72.

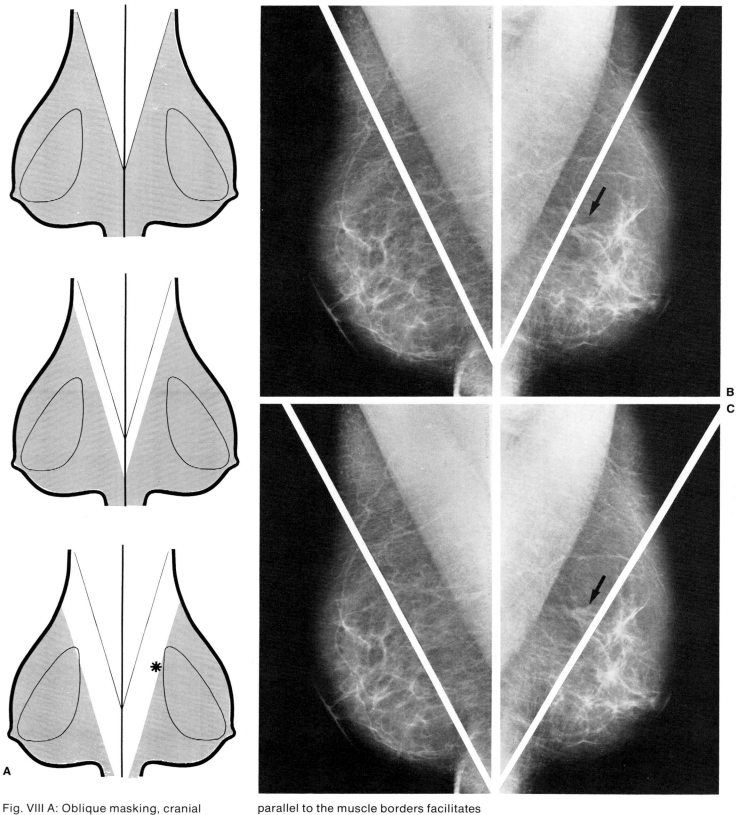

Fig. VIII A: Oblique masking, cranial aspect. Right and left breasts of the medio-lateral oblique (or latero-medial) projections are viewed as shown. The masks are initially placed along the border of the pectoral muscles. Symmetrical stepwise movement keeping the masks parallel to the muscle borders facilitates comparison of the corresponding regions on the mammograms. This is demonstrated in Fig. VIII B (case 74). Oblique masking from the cranial aspect is also very helpful in cases 76, 78, 79, 82.

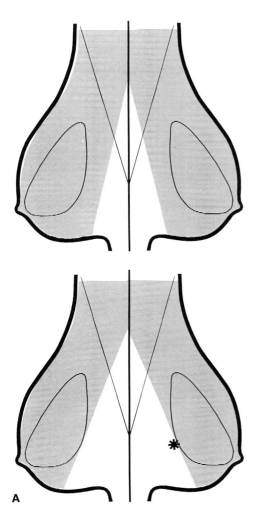

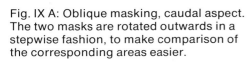

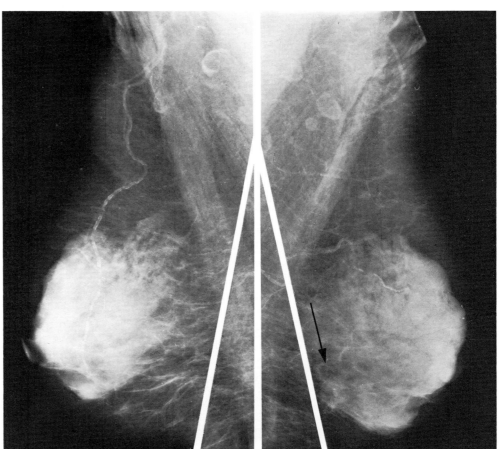

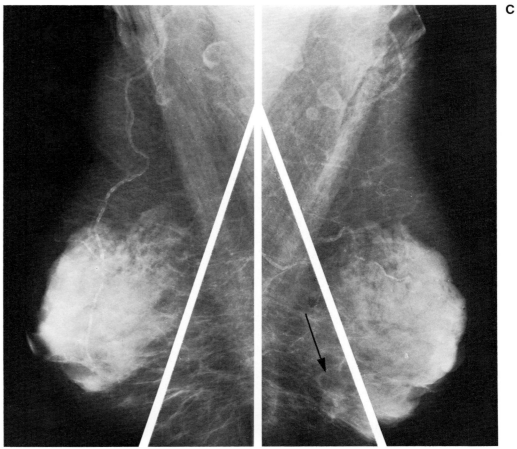

B

C

Fig. IX A: Oblique masking, caudal aspect. The two masks are rotated outwards in a stepwise fashion, to make comparison of the corresponding areas easier.

Fig. IX B, C: Oblique masking, caudal aspect, demonstrated on mammograms.

Fig. X A: Diagrammatic illustration of parenchymal distortion. Asymmetries within the parenchyma, such as localized increases in density or parenchymal distortion, may be the only signs leading to the detection of stellate lesions. Perception of such subtle changes requires careful, systematic comparison of corresponding regions of the parenchyma.

Fig. X B: Right and left mammograms, medio-lateral oblique projections. A stellate lesion is outlined in the right breast.

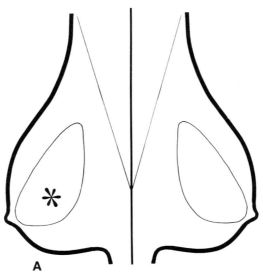

A

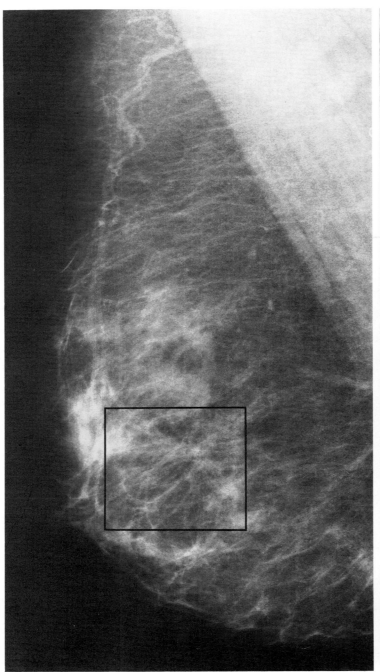
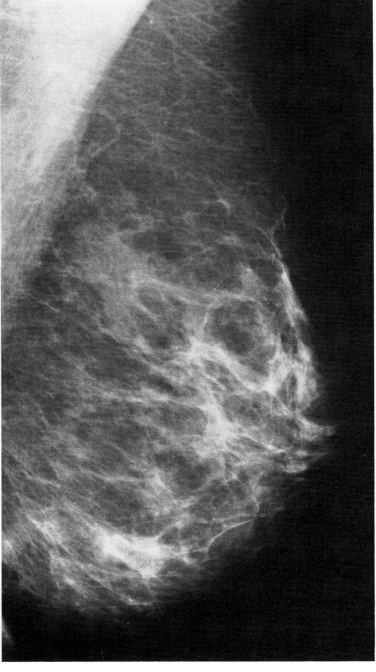

B

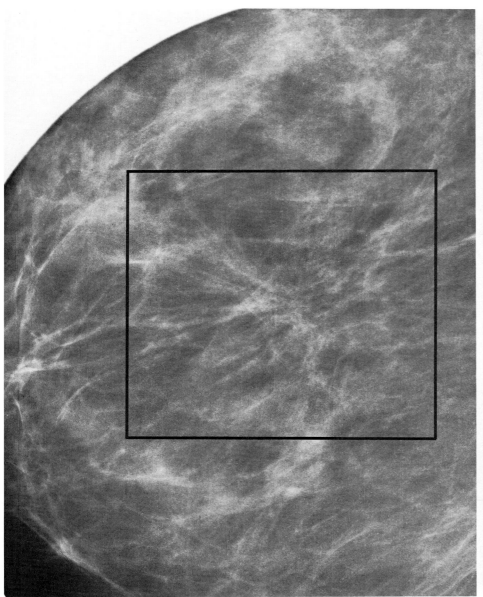 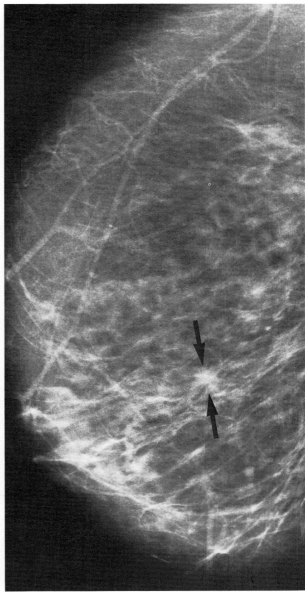

C **D**

Fig. X C: Microfocus magnification view of the stellate lesion provides better analysis of the parenchymal distortion (case 61).

Fig. X D: Small stellate lesions within the parenchyma may be detected only through disturbances of the structure (arrows) (case 70). See also case 77.

Fig. XI A: Schematic demonstration of parenchymal retraction in the cranio-caudal projection, along the lateral border of the parenchyma.

Fig. XI B: Mammographic illustration of parenchymal retraction (arrow) caused by a small carcinoma.

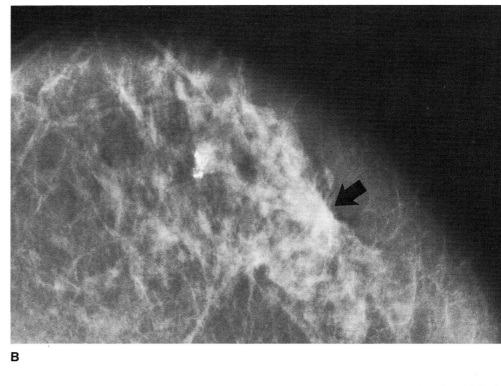

B

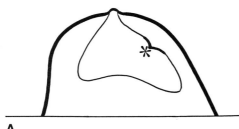

A

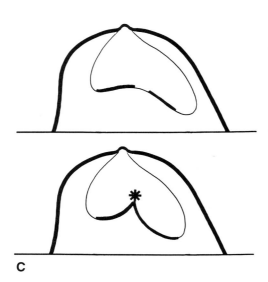

C

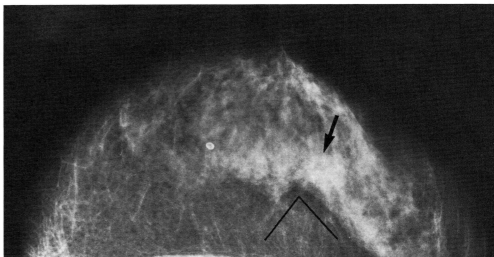

D

Fig. XI C: Retraction along the posterior border of the parenchyma in the cranio-caudal projection gives a special appearance. While the posterior border is normally smooth and usually concave, retraction may lead to a biconvex border resembling the peak of a tent ("tent sign").

Fig. XI D: Mammogram (case 71) demonstrating a tumor (arrow) producing the "tent sign". See case 80 as well.

Fig. XI E–G ▷

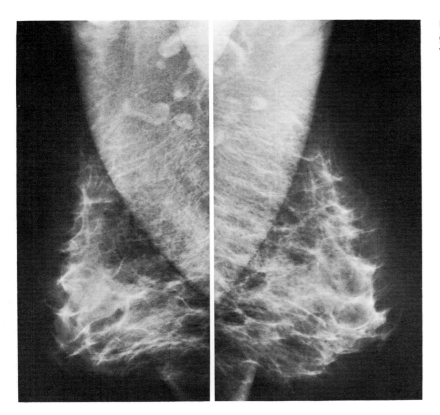

Fig. XI E: 35-year-old woman, right and left mammograms, medio-lateral oblique projections. No tumor is visible. Cranio-caudal projections on Fig. XI F–G.

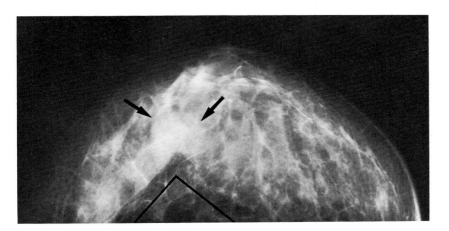

Fig. XI F: Right breast, cranio-caudal projection. Typical "tent sign" (retraction along the posterior border) is seen, caused by a carcinoma (arrows).

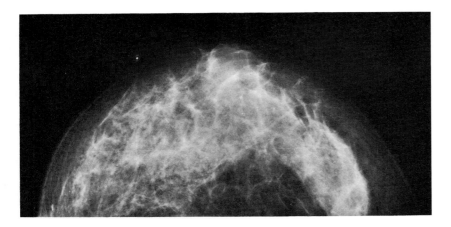

Fig. XI G: Left breast, normal cranio-caudal projection.

Fig. XII A: Detection of parenchymal retraction may lead to the diagnosis of small tumors in dense breasts in which the tumor itself may be hidden. Diagrammatic illustration of retraction of parenchymal contour on the medio-lateral oblique projection.

Fig. XII B: Mammographic demonstration of local retraction of parenchymal contour (arrow). Compare this contour with the corresponding region of the contralateral breast. See also case 80.

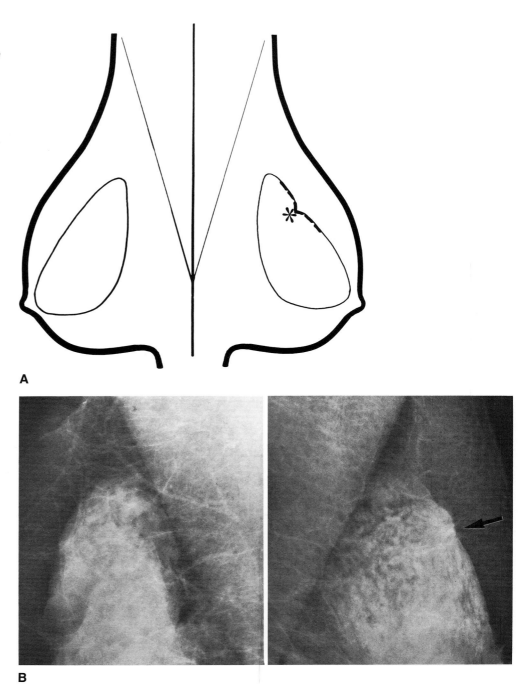

A

B

III. Approach to Mammographic Film Interpretation

When interpreting a mammogram, three steps must be taken:

a) *Determine whether the film is of diagnostic quality* with regard to positioning, exposure and processing. Poor quality mammograms or improper positioning often result in diagnostic errors.

b) *Search for a lesion.* Perception is improved by a systematic survey of the mammograms (see Chapter II). Do not stop looking after you have found one lesion. Remember the other breast, too.

c) *Each detected lesion should be carefully analyzed.*

First, place each lesion into one of the five following classification groups:

I. *Circumscribed lesions* that may be well or poorly outlined, circular, oval or lobulated, solitary or multiple.

II. *Stellate lesions* that are radiating structures with ill-defined periphery.

III. *Calcifications* that may or may not be associated with a tumor. One or more calcifications may constitute the entire radiologic abnormality.

IV. *Thickened skin syndrome* that presents with thickened skin over much or all of the breast, associated with an increased density and a reticular pattern.

V. *Any combination* of two or more of the above lesions.

Second, after finding the proper group, each detected lesion should undergo detailed *analysis* (see Chapters IV–VII).

IV. Circumscribed
Lesions

These may be sharply or poorly outlined; circular, oval or lobulated; solitary or multiple.

If a circumscribed lesion is associated with calcifications, the lesion is analyzed independent of the calcifications. The two analyses are then combined. The following four steps of analysis can rapidly lead to mammographic diagnosis:

Analysis of
1) *Contour*
   a) sharply outlined
      – halo sign
      – capsule
   b) unsharp contour
2) *Density* } primary importance
3) *Form, orientation*
4) *Size* } secondary importance

Signs of Primary Importance in Diagnosing Circumscribed Tumors

A) Halo Sign or Capsule: Present or Absent

The *halo sign* is a narrow radiolucent ring or a segment of a ring around the periphery of a lesion characteristic of benign, growing circumscribed tumors (cases 17, 21, 49, 50, 52, 53, 56). A *capsule* is a thin, curved, radiopaque line that is seen only when it surrounds lesions containing fat (cases 1, 3, 4, 5). Both the halo sign and the capsule are characteristic of benign tumors. Their presence nearly always means that the lesion in question is benign. There are only three rare exceptions, malignant lesions which may have a halo sign:
– intracystic carcinoma,
– papillary carcinoma,
– carcinoma arising within a fibroadenoma (case 103).

Comments

a) Since the diagnostic value of the halo sign is so great, one should search for it with additional projections, in particular with coned-down compression views.
b) The most common circumscribed lesions are cysts and fibroadenomas. An easily visible, obvious halo sign encircling much or all of the lesion is characteristic of a cyst.
   Further differential diagnostic aids: cysts usually occur in women around menopause while fibroadenomas arise in younger women. Cysts are often painful to pressure while fibroadenomas are not.
c) A capsule, when present, has a diagnostic value equal to that of a halo sign.

d) Evaluation of density must always accompany the search for a halo sign or capsule.

B) Density of the Circumscribed Tumor

The evaluation of density is of great importance in diagnosing circumscribed tumors. Density should be evaluated in relation to the surrounding parenchyma, or, in the case of fatty involution, to the nipple.
The tumor, in comparison with the surrounding parenchyma, is either
– radiolucent,
– radiolucent and radiopaque combined,
– low density radiopaque (equal to the surrounding parenchyma),
– high density radiopaque (greater than the surrounding parenchyma).
Once the relative density of the lesion has been determined, the diagnostic choices are limited to the following groups:

Radiolucent Circumscribed Lesions

1) Lipoma (cases 1, 2)
2) Oil cyst (cases 3, 4, 139)
3) Galactocele

Radiolucent and Radiopaque Combined

1) Fibro-adeno-lipoma (cases 5, 6)
2) Galactocele (cases 7, 8)
3) Intramammary lymph node (cases 9, 10, 47, 123)
4) Hematoma (cases 11, 12, 46)

Low Density Radiopaque

The surrounding parenchymal structures (vein, trabeculae, etc.) can be seen "through" the lesion.
1) Fibroadenoma (cases 13, 14, 15, 16, 30, 34, 49, 50, 51)
2) Cyst (cases 17, 18, 19, 52, 53, 56)
Rarer lesions:
3) Giant fibroadenoma (case 21)
4) Atheroma (sebaceous cyst) (case 31)
5) Cavernous hemangioma (cases 23, 151)
6) Papilloma, papillomatosis (cases 27, 48, 127, 128)
7) Wart (cases 24, 25)
8) Abscess
9) Cystosarcoma phylloides (case 26)
10) Papillary carcinoma
11) Mucinous carcinoma (cases 28, 32, 44)
Note: These malignant lesions may lead to difficulties in diagnosis.

High Density Radiopaque

These are more dense than the surrounding parenchyma. Structures such as veins, trabeculae, etc. cannot be seen "through" the dense lesion.
1) Carcinoma (e.g. medullary, solid) (cases 29, 33, 41, 54)
2) Sarcoma
3) Metastases to the breast (cases 36, 40)
4) Cystosarcoma phylloides (case 37)
5) Cyst (case 20)
6) Abscess (cases 38, 42)
7) Hematoma
8) Enlarged lymph nodes (lymphoma, leukemia, rheumatoid arthritis, metastases) (cases 43, 45)
9) Atheroma (sebaceous cyst) (case 22).
Note: All radiolucent, all radiolucent and radiopaque combined, and most low density radiopaque lesions are benign.

Signs of Secondary Importance in Diagnosing Circumscribed Lesions

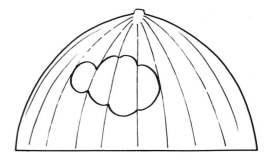

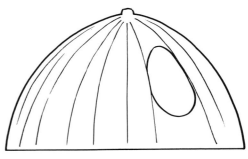

These serve as confirmation of diagnoses which should have already been made on the basis of contour and density analysis.

A) Form and Orientation of the Circumscribed Lesions

(Fig. XIII)

A *cyst* is generally spherical or ovoid with smooth borders. Its orientation, when elongated, is usually in the direction of the nipple following the trabecular structure of the breast (cases 53, 56).

A *solid tumor* (e.g. fibroadenoma, carcinoma) may be smooth or lobulated. Its orientation is random as it does not tend to be aligned along the trabecular structure of the breast (cases 49, 54).

B) Size

Circumscribed lesions can be grouped into three categories according to size, providing for a certain degree of differential diagnosis.

Very Large Circumscribed Lesions (> 5 cm)

Few breast tumors grow this large; they displace much of the breast tissue. The diagnoses can be limited to the following list:

a) **Radiolucent**
1) Lipoma (case 1)

b) **Radiolucent and radiopaque combined**
1) Fibro-adeno-lipoma (cases 5, 6)

c) **Radiopaque**
Low density radiopaque:
1) Giant fibroadenoma (case 21)
2) Cyst (cases 17, 56)
3) Cystosarcoma phylloides (case 26)
4) Mucinous carcinoma (case 32)
High density radiopaque:
1) Carcinoma (case 54)
2) Sarcoma
3) Cystosarcoma phylloides (case 37)

4) Cyst
5) Abscess (cases 38, 42)
6) Lymph nodes (lymphoma, leukemia, metastases)

Intermediate Sized Circumscribed Lesions (on the order of 3−5 cm)

a) **Radiolucent**
1) Lipoma
2) Oil cyst (case 139)

b) **Radiolucent and radiopaque combined**
1) Fibro-adeno-lipoma
2) Hematoma (case 46)

c) **Radiopaque**
Low density radiopaque:
1) Fibroadenoma (cases 13, 49, 50, 55)
2) Cyst (cases 39, 52)
3) Atheroma (sebaceous cyst)
4) Mucinous carcinoma, which may cause diagnostic difficulties
High density radiopaque:
1) Carcinoma
2) Sarcoma
3) Metastases to the breast (case 40)
4) Cystosarcoma phylloides
5) Abscess
6) Cyst (case 20)
7) Atheroma (sebaceous cyst) (case 22)
8) Lymph nodes (lymphoma, leukemia, rheumatoid arthritis, metastases) (cases 43, 45)

Smaller Circumscribed Lesions (< 3 cm)

a) **Radiolucent**
1) Lipoma (case 2)
2) Oil cyst (cases 3, 4)
3) Galactocele

b) **Radiolucent and radiopaque combined**
1) Galactocele (cases 7, 8)
2) Intramammary lymph node (cases 9, 10, 47, 123)
3) Hematoma (cases 11, 12)
4) Fibro-adeno-lipoma (rare when small)

c) **Radiopaque**
Low density radiopaque:
1) Fibroadenoma (cases 14, 15, 16, 30, 34, 51)
2) Cyst (cases 18, 19, 53)
Rarer lesions:
3) Atheroma (sebaceous cyst) (case 31)
4) Intramammary lymph node
5) Papilloma, Papillomatosis (cases 127, 128)
6) Hemangioma (case 23)
7) Carcinoma, most frequently mucinous (cases 28, 44) or papillary
8) Wart (cases 24, 25)
High density radiopaque:
1) Carcinoma (cases 29, 33)
2) Metastasis to the breast (case 36)
3) Lymph nodes (metastases, leukemia, lymphoma, rheumatoid arthritis)

Fig. XIII A & B: The orientation of solid tumors (fibroadenoma, carcinoma, etc.) is usually random as they tend not to be aligned along the trabecular structure of the breast (A), while the trabecular structure can influence the orientation of a cyst (B).

Strategy

After the four steps of analysis (contour, density, form and orientation, and size), one should have formed an opinion whether the lesion is benign or malignant. Fine needle puncture of the circumscribed lesion may provide considerable help in deciding whether surgical biopsy is necessary.

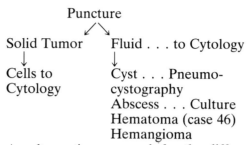

Puncture

Solid Tumor   Fluid . . . to Cytology

Cells to   Cyst . . . Pneumo-
Cytology   cystography
              Abscess . . . Culture
              Hematoma (case 46)
              Hemangioma

An alternative approach for the differentiation of cystic from solid tumors is the use of breast sonography, which is highly accurate for this purpose. This method is especially useful with the non-palpable, benign-appearing radiopaque masses, which otherwise need to be punctured under mammographic guidance.

When ultrasonography and/or puncture demonstrate that the non-palpable circumscribed lesion is non-cystic, contour analysis becomes particularly important. Lesions with unsharp borders should be biopsied after preoperative localization (ref. 16).

Many circumscribed lesions do not require biopsy. The most striking example of this is a cyst, of which 95% can be cured by pneumocystography alone (ref. 24, 39, 45).

Mammographic diagnosis of lipomas, fibro-adeno-lipomas, oil cysts, intramammary lymph nodes and most of the fibroadenomas is highly reliable, especially in combination with aspiration cytology. Since so many circumscribed lesions are found in a screening program, it is necessary to diagnose most of them definitively by mammography and fine needle puncture, referring only a fraction of them to surgical biopsy.

Practice in Analyzing Circumscribed Tumors

(Cases 1–56)

1

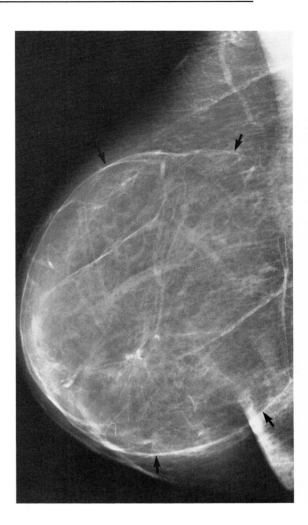

Age 85. First screening study, asymptomatic.

Physical Examination

A huge, soft, round tumor is palpable in the right breast.

Mammography

Fig. 1: Right breast, medio-lateral oblique projection. A huge, encapsulated lesion occupies the whole breast. There are central calcifications.

Analysis

Form: circumscribed, circular
Contour: sharp; a capsule surrounds the lesion
Density: radiolucent
Size: huge, 12 × 12 cm

Conclusion

The only huge radiolucent breast tumor is a lipoma.

Comment

The central, ring-like and irregular calcifications, some with a radiolucent center, appear to be the result of fat necrosis (see page 172).

2

Age 34, referred for evaluation of breast pain.

Physical Examination

No palpable tumor.

Mammography

Fig. 2: Right breast, medio-lateral oblique projection. There is a solitary lesion 5 cm from the nipple in the upper medial quadrant. No associated calcifications.

Analysis

Form: circumcribed, oval
Contour: sharply outlined; the lesion is encapsulated
Density: radiolucent
Size: 20 × 15 mm

Conclusion

The density is the factor determining the mammographic diagnosis of a lipoma.

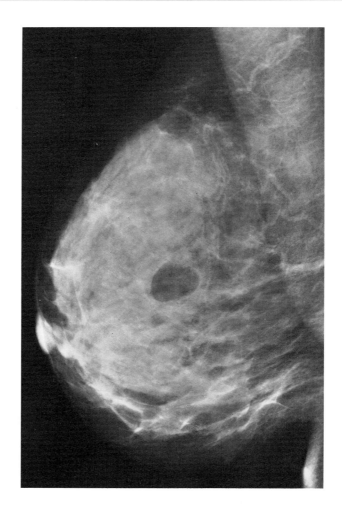

3

A 58-year-old woman previously operated for a benign lesion in the right breast.

Mammography

Fig. 3 A & B: Right breast, mediolateral oblique projection. An oval-shaped tumor is seen centrally in the breast without associated calcifications. A scar is seen between the lesion and the skin (Fig. 3 B, arrow).

Analysis

Form: circumscribed, oval
Contour: sharp, no halo sign but a definite capsule
Density: radiolucent
Size: 15 × 12 mm

Conclusion

The history of surgical biopsy at this site combined with the mammographic appearance is typical for an oil cyst (see page 172).

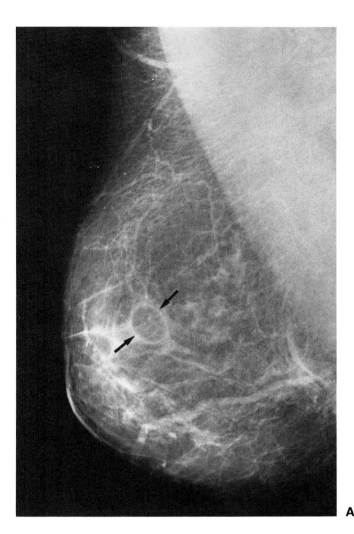

A

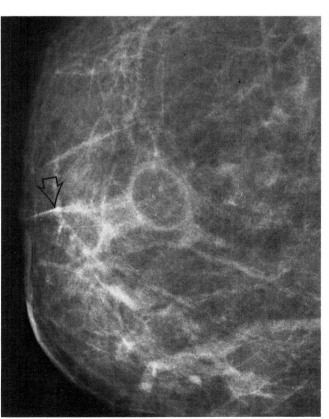

B

4

A 48-year-old woman with a history of excisional biopsy in the retro-areolar region.

Mammography

Fig. 4: Detailed view of the medio-lateral oblique projection of the left breast. There is a partly calcified retromammillary tumor.

Analysis

Form: circumscribed, circular
Contour: sharp
Density: radiolucent
Size: 10 × 10 mm

Comment

There are also shell-like calcifications in the wall of the lesion.

Conclusion

There are three possible circumscribed, radiolucent lesions, all benign (page 18). In this case, the history of biopsy leads to the diagnosis of an oil cyst. With a partially calcified capsule, it is known as liponecrosis macrocystica calcificans (page 172).

Note

There are many ring-like calcifications near the oil cyst. These represent liponecrosis microcystica calcificans.

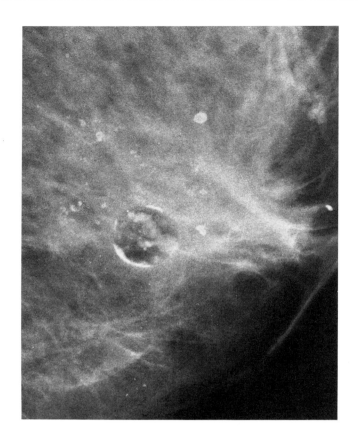

5

Right breast, cranio-caudal projection. There is a large, centrally-located tumor with no associated calcifications (Fig. 5).

Analysis

Form: circumscribed, oval
Contour: sharp, capsule seen
Density: radiolucent and radiopaque combined
Size: 6 × 6 cm

Conclusion

Benign tumor. A large, encapsulated tumor with mixed density is characteristic of a fibro-adeno-lipoma.

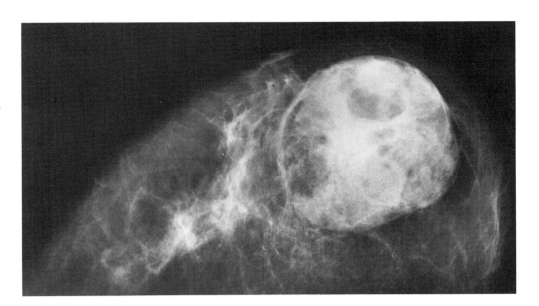

6

Left breast, medio-lateral oblique projection. A large tumor fills in the central portion of the breast (Fig. 6).

Analysis

Form: circumscribed, oval
Contour: sharply outlined, encapsulated; a halo sign is seen along the anterior border
Density: radiopaque and radiolucent combined (predominantly glandular components)
Size: 7 × 4 cm

Conclusion

Typical mammographic appearance of a fibro-adeno-lipoma, which is a huge, encapsulated, benign lesion consisting of a mixture of fat and glandular structures.

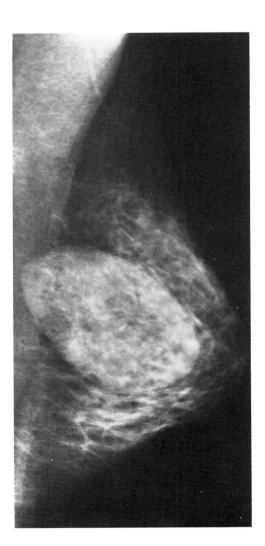

7

This 28-year-old woman noted a lump in her right breast during nursing.

Mammography

Fig. 7 A: Left breast, cranio-caudal projection.
Fig. 7 B: Detailed view of the retroareolar region. A tumor with mixed density is seen (arrow).

Analysis

Form: circumscribed, lobulated
Contour: sharply defined
Density: radiolucent and radiopaque combined
Size: 12 × 10 mm

Differential Diagnosis

There are four possible diagnostic choices for a tumor of mixed density. The history points to a galactocele. The small size helps to differentiate it from a fibro-adeno-lipoma which is practically always large. The absence of trauma or previous breast surgery helps to exclude a hematoma or oil cyst.

Conclusion

The mammographic diagnosis is a benign tumor, as are all tumors with combined radiolucent and radiopaque densities (page 18).
The history and mammographic appearance are consistent with a *galactocele,* which is a milk-filled cyst with a high fat content appearing at the time of lactation.

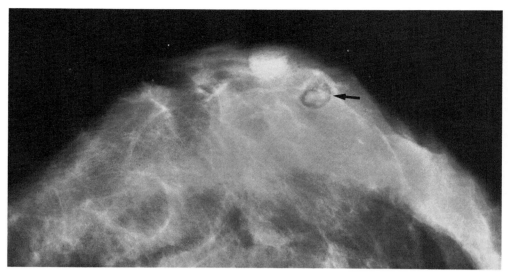

A

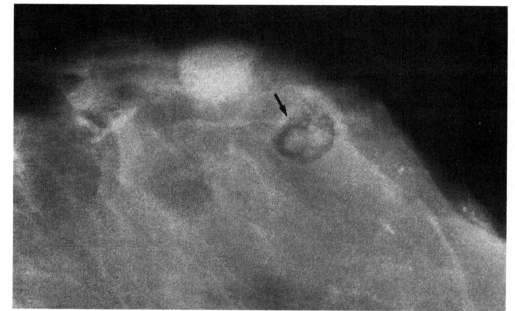

B

8

This 42-year-old woman noted a mass in her breast two months following the completion of nursing.

Mammography

Fig. 8 A: Right breast, medio-lateral oblique projection. A tumor is seen 7 cm from the nipple.
Fig. 8 B: Enlarged view of the tumor.

Analysis

Form: circumscribed, oval
Contour: sharply defined
Density: radiolucent and radiopaque combined
Size: 25 × 20 mm

Conclusion

The history and mammographic appearance are typical of a galactocele.

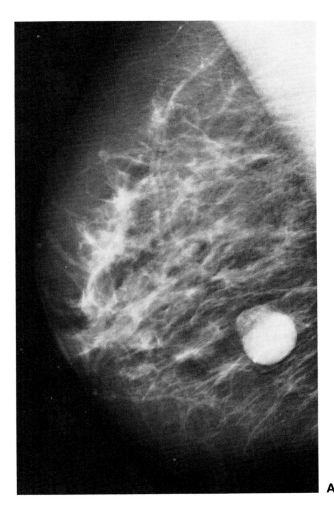

A

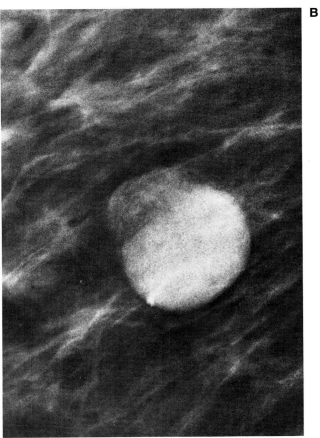

B

9

Age 80. First screening examination, asymptomatic.

Physical Examination

A very soft, freely movable superficial lesion is palpable in the upper outer quadrant of the left breast, clinically benign.

Mammography

Fig. 9 A: Left breast, medio-lateral oblique projection. A solitary lesion is seen in the upper outer quadrant.
Fig. 9 B: An enlarged view of the lesion.

Analysis

Form: circumscribed, lobulated
Contour: mostly sharp; no halo sign is seen
Density: radiolucent and radiopaque combined
Size: 15 × 10 mm

Conclusion

This is one of the four circumscribed lesions with combined radiolucent and radiopaque densities (page 18), all of which are benign. Further differentiation can be made as follows: a fibro-adeno-lipoma is practically always huge, a galactocele is associated with nursing, and a hematoma is associated with trauma. This lesion is an intra-mammary lymph node with a typical central radiolucency corresponding to the hilus.

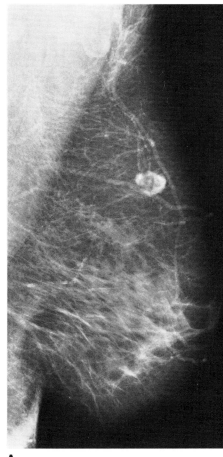

A

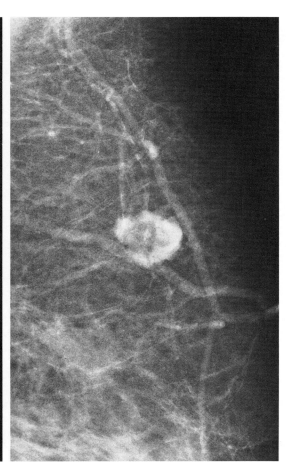

B

10

First screening examination of this 64-year-old asymptomatic woman.

Physical Examination

No palpable tumor.

Mammography

Fig. 10 A: Right breast, medio-lateral oblique projection. Small circumscribed lesion is seen in the upper outer quadrant. No associated calcifications.

Fig. 10 B: Enlarged view of the lesion.

Analysis

Form: circumscribed, oval
Contour: sharply outlined
Density: radiopaque and radiolucent combined
Size: 6 × 5 mm

Conclusion

The mixed density is crucial in classifying this finding: small intramammary lymph node. The central radiolucent area corresponds to the hilus.

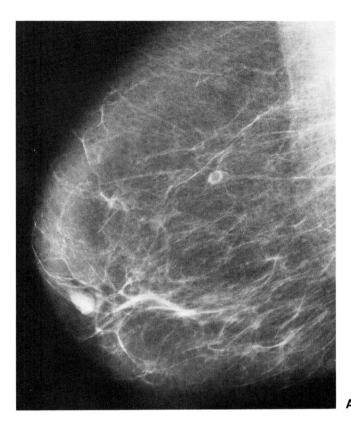

A

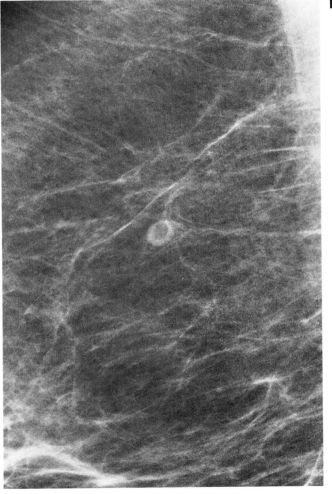

B

11

Age 65. Trauma to the right breast eight days earlier.

Mammography

Fig. 11 A: Right breast, cranio-caudal projection. A tumor is seen 4 cm from the nipple. No associated calcifications.
Fig. 11 B: Enlarged view of the tumor.

Comment

There are four differential diagnostic choices for a circumscribed lesion with mixed density. In this case the history of recent trauma leads to the diagnosis of a hematoma.

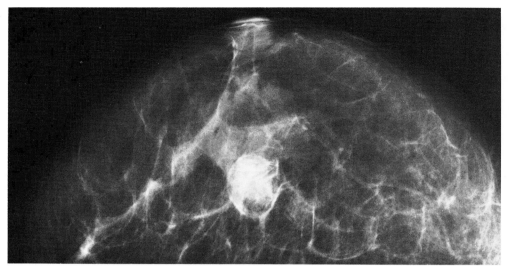

A

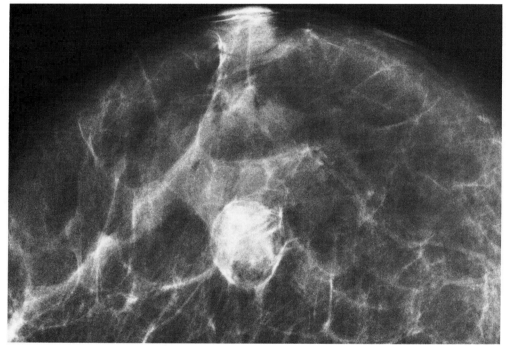

B

12

Age 67. The patient experienced trauma to the right breast two weeks earlier. In addition to a superficial hematoma she noted a lump.

Mammography

Fig. 12 A & B: Right breast, medio-lateral oblique and cranio-caudal projections. Superficial solitary tumor in the lower lateral quadrant. No associated calcifications.
Fig. 12 C: Enlarged view of the tumor.

Analysis

Form: circumscribed, oval
Contour: sharply outlined
Density: radiopaque and radiolucent combined; the radiolucent area is small and is best seen on the enlarged view (arrow)
Size: 20 × 15 mm

Conclusion

Both history and mammographic appearance indicate a hematoma. This will eventually develop into an oil cyst.

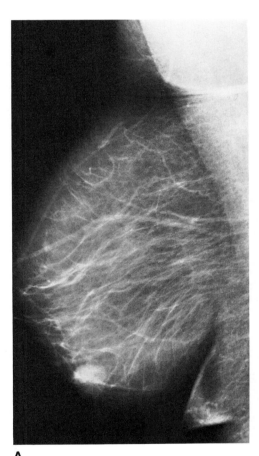

A

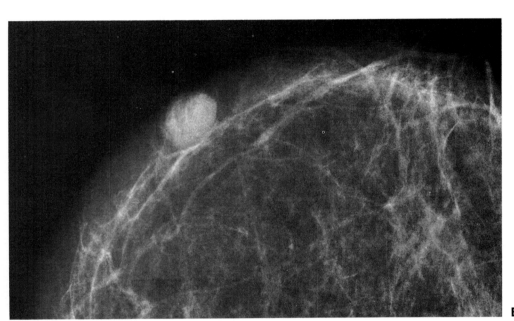

B

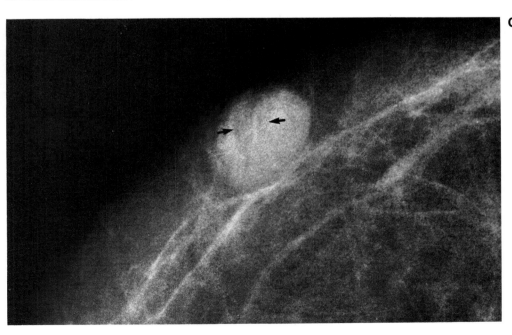

C

13

Age 52. First screening examination, asymptomatic.

Physical Examination

3 cm, firm, freely movable retro-areolar tumor. Inverted nipple, no skin changes. Clinically benign.

Mammography

Fig. 13 A & B: Right breast, medio-lateral oblique and cranio-caudal projections. There is a circumscribed retroareolar tumor with no associated calcifications. A smaller tumor is seen in the upper outer quadrant 6 cm from the nipple.

Analysis

Form: circumscribed, oval, lobulated
Contour: sharply outlined
Density: low density radiopaque
Size: 30 × 15 mm

Comment

When a circumscribed lesion is low density radiopaque on the mammogram, *contour analysis* will be decisive. The halo sign or a sharp contour completely surrounding the lesion indicates that it is benign.

When a circumscribed lesion is either radiolucent or radiolucent and radiopaque combined on the mammogram, *density analysis* is decisive in determining that it is benign.

Conclusion

Mammographically benign tumor. The smaller lesion, 6 cm from the nipple, is also a sharply outlined, low density lobulated tumor. Mammographically benign.

Histology

Two fibroadenomas.

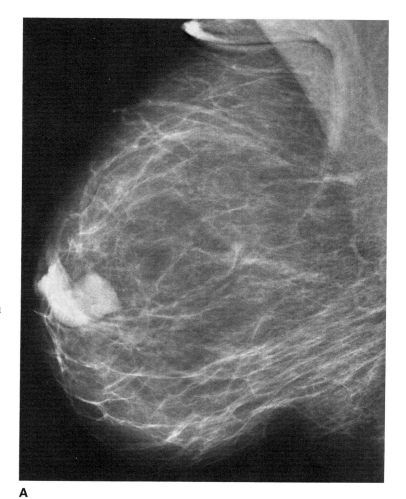

A

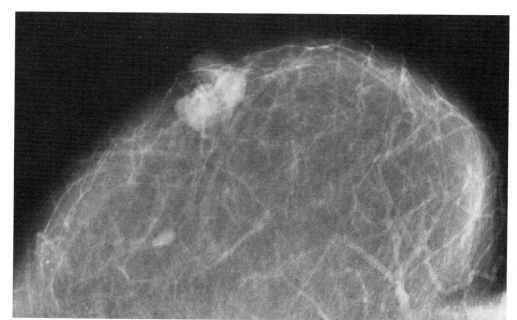

B

14

Age 42. First screening examination, asymptomatic.

Physical Examination

2 cm tumor in the upper inner quadrant of the right breast, clinically benign.

Mammography

Fig. 14 A: Right breast, medio-lateral oblique projection. There is a tumor with no associated calcifications 6 cm from the nipple in the upper half of the breast.

Fig. 14 B & C: Enlarged views of the tumor in the medio-lateral and craniocaudal projections.

Analysis

Form: circumscribed, oval, lobulated
Contour: mostly sharp, but there are many disturbing overlying parenchymal shadows
Density: low density radiopaque; a superimposed vessel and parenchyma can be clearly seen
Size: 2 × 2 cm

Conclusion

Tumor probably benign.

Histology

Fibroadenoma.

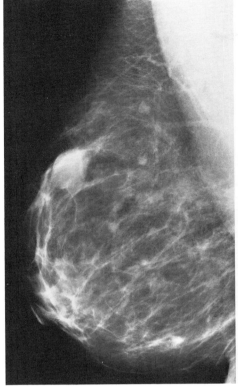
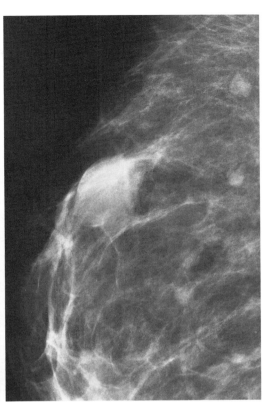

A   B

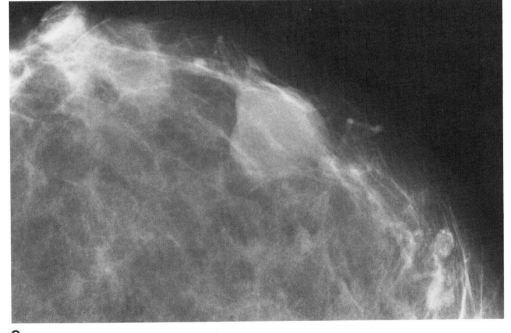

C

15

Asymptomatic 75-year-old woman, first screening study.

Physical Examination

Approximately 2 cm freely movable tumor in the lower outer quadrant of the right breast. No skin changes.

Mammography

Fig. 15 A & B: Right breast, cranio-caudal and medio-lateral oblique projections. Circumscribed tumor 7 cm from the nipple in the lower outer quadrant. No associated calcifications. Fig. 15 C & D: Enlarged views of the tumor in the cranio-caudal and medio-lateral oblique projections. A partially calcified artery is seen to overly the tumor in Fig. D.

Analysis

Form: circumscribed, oval
Contour: mostly unsharp; no definite halo sign
Density: low density radiopaque
Size: 20 × 15 mm

Conclusion

A tumor with unsharp borders in a 75-year-old woman raises the suspicion of malignancy.

Cytology

Cells suspicious for malignancy.

Histology

Fibroadenoma.

Comment

In a radiopaque circumscribed tumor, the absence of a halo sign or a sharply outlined contour around the entire lesion makes biopsy mandatory.

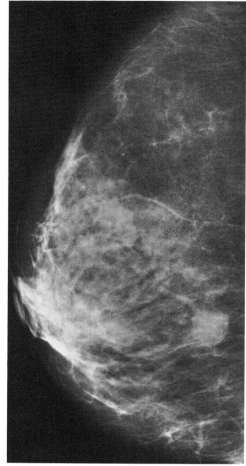

A

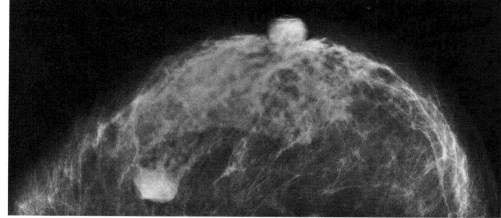

B

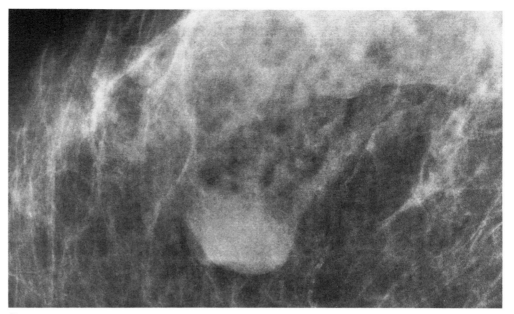

C

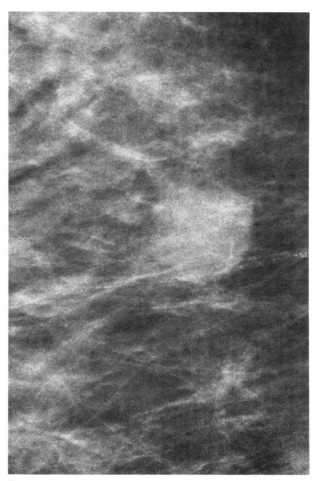

D

16

Age 33, referred for a self-detected tumor in the right breast.

Mammography

Fig. 16 A & B: Right breast, medio-lateral oblique and cranio-caudal projections.
Fig. 16 C: Coned-down compression view in the cranio-caudal projection, photographic enlargement.
A solitary tumor without associated calcifications is seen in the upper outer quadrant of the breast.

Analysis

Form: circumscribed, oval
Contour: only the posterior border is sharply outlined; there is a halo sign present on the compression view (arrows)
Density: low density radiopaque, equal to the parenchyma
Size: 15 × 15 mm

Conclusion

Mammographically benign tumor.

Histology

Fibroadenoma.

Comment

The halo sign detected on the coned-down view is crucial in determining the benign nature of this lesion. The unsharp borders made biopsy necessary.

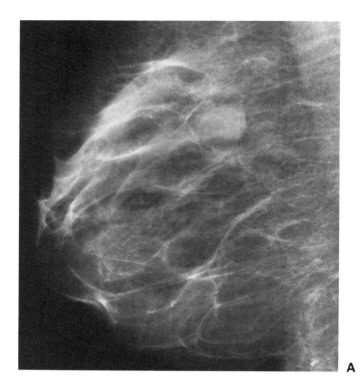

A

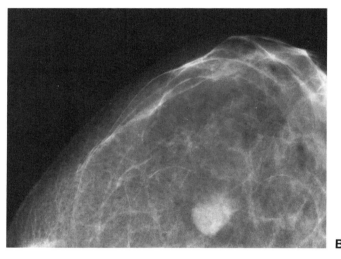

B

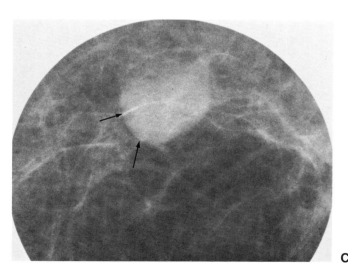

C

17

Age 50. First screening examination. The patient was aware of a tumor in her left breast but did not seek medical advice.

Physical Examination

Tender, 5 cm, clinically benign retroareolar lesion.

Mammography

Fig. 17 A: Right breast, detailed view of the cranio-caudal projection. There is a solitary retroareolar tumor with no associated calcifications.

Analysis

Form: circumscribed, oval
Contour: extensive halo sign
Density: low density radiopaque
Size: 5 × 5 cm

Conclusion

Mammographically benign tumor, typical appearance of a cyst.
Fig. 17 B: Pneumocystogram. Simple cyst, no intracystic tumor.

Comment

The halo sign may be extensive in cysts whereas in fibroadenomas the halo sign, when present, is usually short and may be difficult to demonstrate. Puncture of the circumscribed tumor helps in differentiating a solid tumor from a cyst.

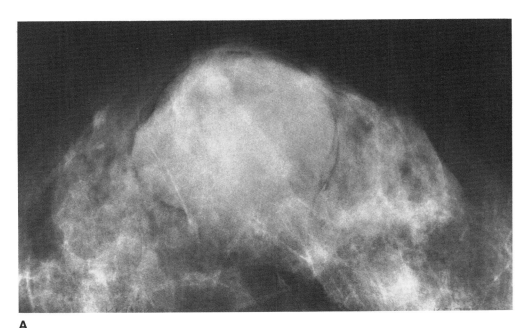

A

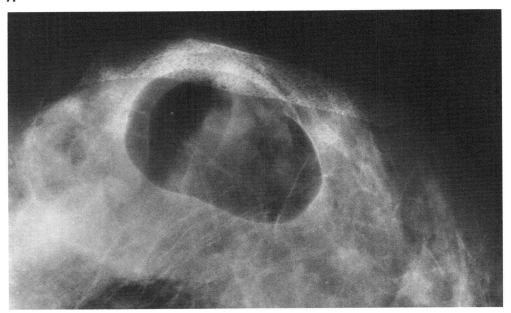

B

18

Age 72. First screening study, asymptomatic.

Physical Examination

Retroareolar tumor, 3 cm diameter, clinically benign.

Mammography

Fig. 18 A & B: Left breast, mediolateral oblique and cranio-caudal projections. Solitary circumscribed retroareolar tumor. No associated calcifications.

Fig. 18 C: Microfocus magnification view, cranio-caudal projection.

Analysis

Form: circumscribed, lobulated
Contour: a halo sign is seen along the anterior border (arrows); overlying parenchyma obscures the posterior border
Density: parenchymal structures can be seen through the tumor
Size: 3 × 2 cm

Conclusion

Mammographically benign tumor.

Puncture and Pneumocystography

(Fig. 18 D)

Cranio-caudal projection. Simple cyst with no intracystic tumor. Air in the needle track.

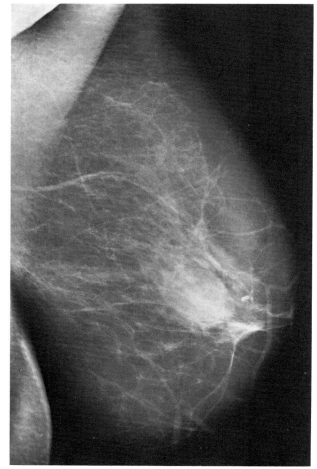

A

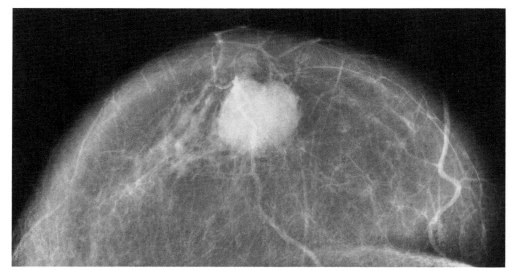

B

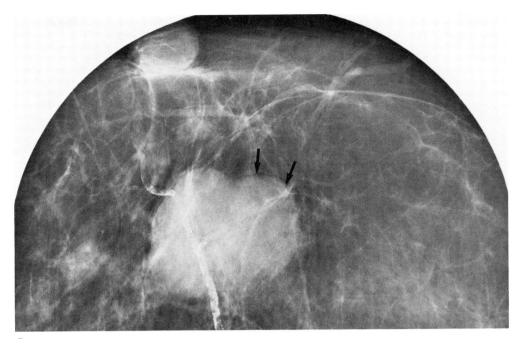

C

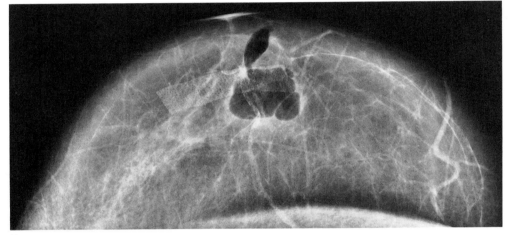

D

19

Asymptomatic, 68-year-old woman, first screening study.

Physical Examination

No palpable tumor.

Mammography

Fig. 19 A & B: Right breast, medio-lateral oblique and cranio-caudal projections. A small solitary tumor with no associated calcifications is seen in the upper outer quadrant.
Fig. 19 C & D: Microfocus magnification views, medio-lateral and cranio-caudal projections.

Analysis

Form: circumscribed, irregular
Contour: partially sharp, partially poorly defined
Density: low density radiopaque; a vein can be seen through the tumor (Fig. 19 D).
Size: 6 × 5 mm

Conclusion

Although the lesion is of low density, the lack of a halo sign and the partially unsharp borders raise the suspicion of malignancy in this 68-year-old woman.

Histology

Simple cyst, no evidence of malignancy.

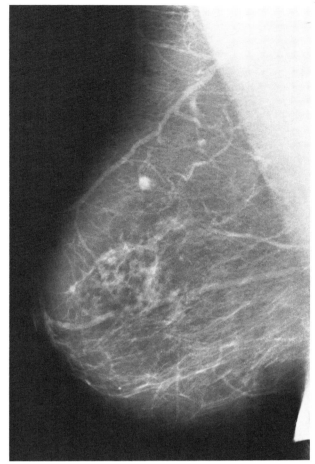

A

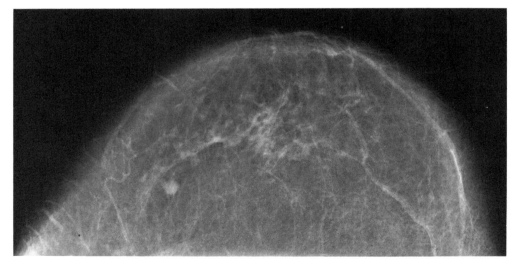

B

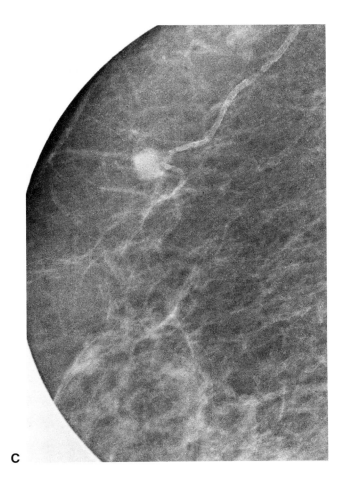

C

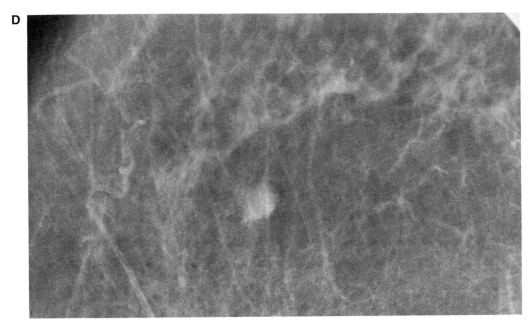

D

20

54-year-old woman, referred for a lump in the right breast, first noted one week earlier.

Physical Examination

Freely movable, hard lump in the lateral portion of the right breast, clinically suspicious for malignancy.

Mammography

Fig. 20 A & B: Right breast, mediolateral oblique and cranio-caudal projections. Solitary circumscribed tumor with no associated calcifications.

Analysis

Form: circumscribed, lobulated
Contour: segments of a halo sign; overlying parenchyma obscures portions of the border
Density: high density radiopaque
Size: 5 × 3 cm

Conclusion

The presence of halo sign suggests that the tumor is benign. The high density makes a cyst, cystosarcoma phylloides or an intracystic tumor all diagnostic possibilities. Puncture is necessary for diagnosis.
Fig. 20 C : Pneumocystogram. Simple cyst, no intracystic tumor.

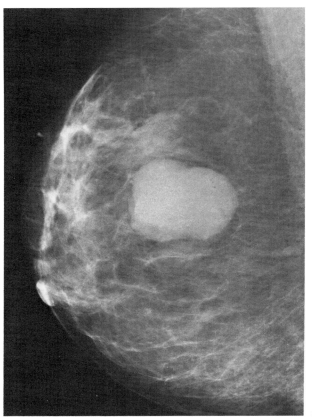

A

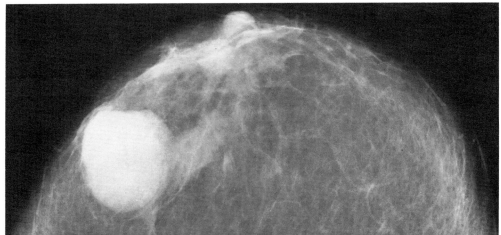

B

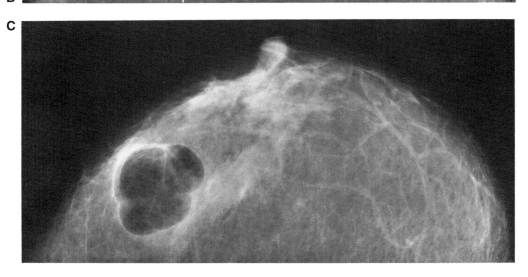

C

21

Age 21. The patient detected a large tumor in her left breast.

Physical Examination

Huge, approximately 10 cm, firm but movable tumor filling most of the left breast.

Mammography

Fig. 21: Left breast, medio-lateral oblique projection.

Analysis

Form: circumscribed, oval
Contour: sharply outlined; extensive halo sign
Density: low density radiopaque, equal to parenchyma
Size: 11 × 8 cm

Conclusion

Large benign tumor. In a patient this young the description is characteristic of a giant fibroadenoma.

Histology

Giant fibroadenoma.

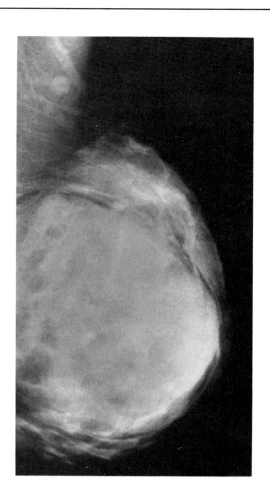

22

67-year-old woman, first noted a tumor in her right breast many years ago but had not sought medical help. First screening examination.

Mammography

Fig. 22 A & B: Right breast, medio-lateral oblique and cranio-caudal projections. A solitary tumor is located in the upper outer quadrant, immediately under the skin. No associated calcifications.

Analysis

Form: circumscribed, oval
Contour: sharply outlined; an air pocket adjacent to this protruding tumor (Fig. 22 A) mimics the halo sign
Size: 3 × 3 cm
Location: intra- and subcutaneous; the overlying skin is not thickened.

Conclusion

Mammographically a typical benign tumor. Clinical examination reveals an atheroma (sebaceous cyst).

Histology

Atheroma (sebaceous cyst).

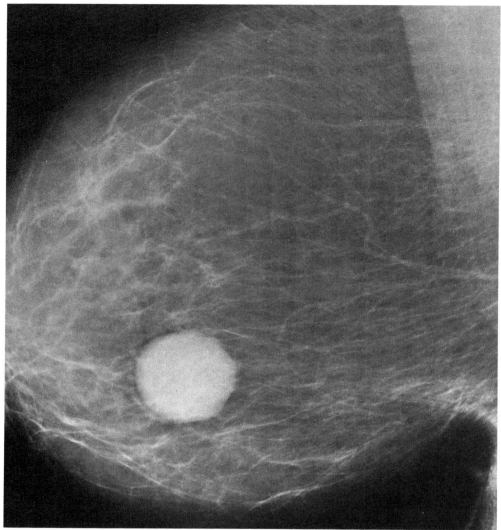

A

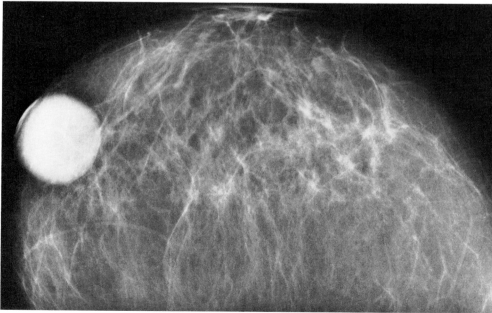

B

23

Asymptomatic 63-year-old woman. First screening study.

Physical Examination

No palpable tumor.

Mammography

Fig. 23 A: Left breast, medio-lateral oblique projection. A solitary tumor is located in the lower half of the breast.
Fig. 23 B & C: Microfocus magnification views in the medio-lateral oblique and cranio-caudal projections. Numerous microcalcifications are seen in the tumor.

Analysis of the Tumor

Form: circumscribed, round, lobulated
Contour: sharply outlined
Density: low density radiopaque
Size: 12 × 15 mm

Analysis of the Calcifications

Form: ovoid and elongate, smooth bordered
Density: high, uniform
Size: small, variable
Distribution: within the tumor

Conclusion

Mammographically benign tumor, containing calcifications of varying size and form.

Histology

Cavernous hemangioma.

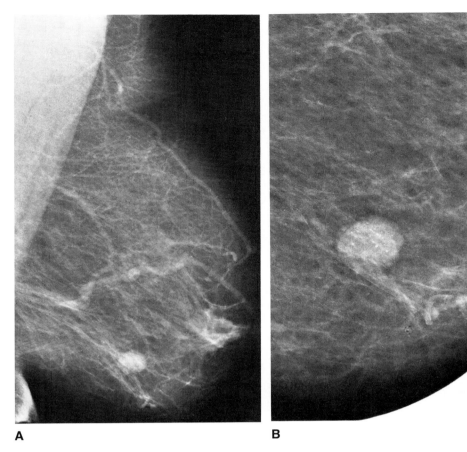

A   B

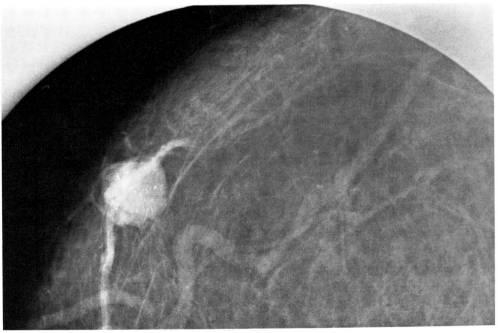

C

24 & 25

Fig. 24 & 25: Two cases of warts. Most warts give a typical mammographic appearance. The borders are sharply outlined with a multilobulated contour. The air outlining the fine, papillary surface emphasizes its structure.

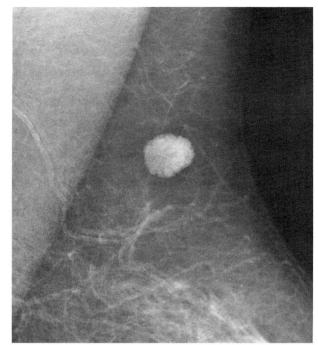

24

25

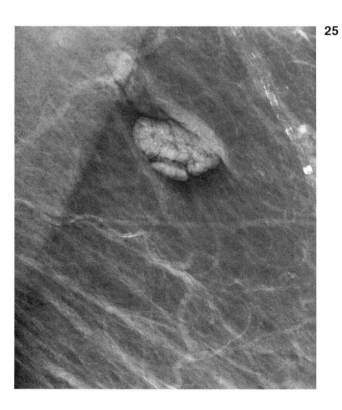

26

Asymptomatic 47-year-old woman.
First screening examination.

Physical Examination

A freely movable tumor, 7 × 6 cm,
fills the upper outer quadrant of the
left breast. No skin retraction.

Mammography

Fig. 26 A & B: Left breast, medio-
lateral oblique and cranio-caudal projections. A large tumor is seen in the
upper outer quadrant associated with
coarse calcifications.

Analysis of the Tumor

Form: circumscribed, oval
Contour: sharply outlined; extensive
halo sign in Fig. 26 A
Density: Equal to the parenchyma
Size: 7 × 6 cm

Analysis of the Calcifications

Coarse, high density, mammographically benign type.

Comment

Huge sharply outlined radiopaque
tumors in women around menopausal
age are characteristic of cystosarcoma
phylloides or, rarely, cysts. In this case
the calcifications indicate the diagnosis
of cystosarcoma phylloides, which is a
large variant of fibroadenoma. It typically occurs around menopause.
Sarcoma or carcinoma may rarely arise
within this tumor.

Histology

Cystosarcoma phylloides.

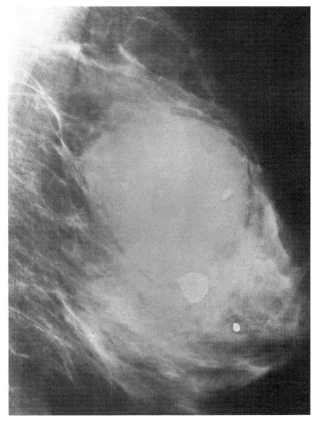

A

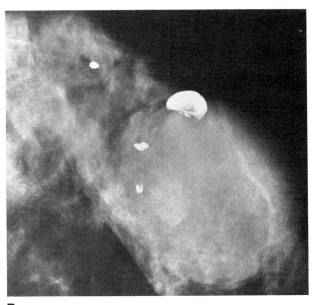

B

27

73-year-old woman, first felt a tender mass behind the left areola one week earlier.

Mammography

Fig. 27 A & B: Right breast, medio-lateral oblique and cranio-caudal projections. The are several retroareolar tumors, the largest containing a single, benign-type calcification.

Analysis

Form: circumscribed, round and oval
Contour: sharply defined, except for the one with the calcification
Density: low density radiopaque; a vein is well seen superimposed over the tumors (Fig. 27 B).
Size: 0.5–2.0 cm
Location: retroareolar

Conclusion

The tumors with sharp borders and low density are mammographically benign, but the mammographic diagnosis of the largest tumor is uncertain. Blood was expressed from the nipple at mammography. Galactography may assist in the diagnosis.

Galactography

(cranio-caudal projection, Fig. 27 C)

A dilated duct leads to the tumors which are seen as intraductal filling defects. Radiologic diagnosis: papillomatosis (see ref. 55).

Histology

Intraductal papillomatosis. No evidence of malignancy.

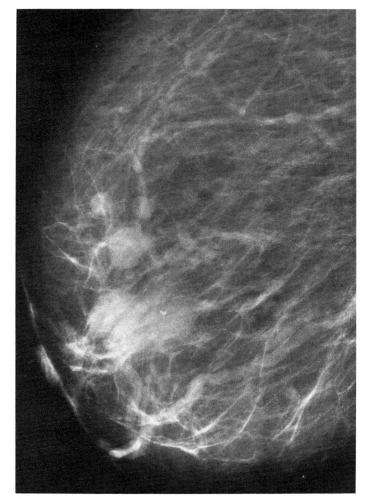

A

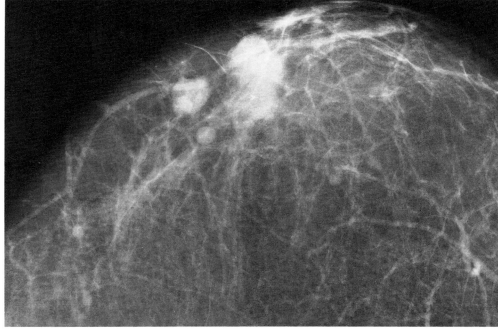

B

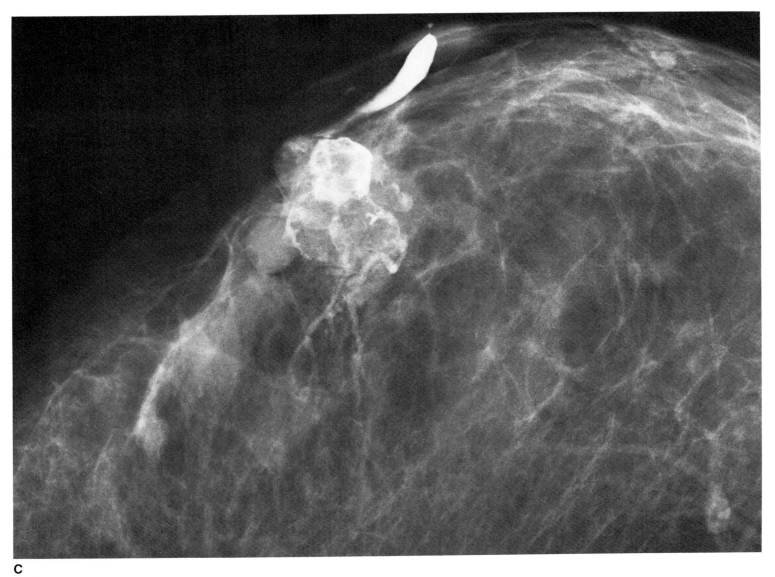

c

28

Asymptomatic 80-year-old woman. First screening study.

Mammography

Fig. 28 A: Right breast, medio-lateral oblique projection. Normal mammogram.
Seven months later the patient felt a lump in the lower half of the right breast.

Repeat Mammography

Fig. 28 B: Right breast, medio-lateral oblique projection. Four cm from the nipple (arrows) there is an ill-defined tumor, not present in the previous study.
Fig. 28 C: Microfocus magnification view in the medio-lateral oblique projection. The tumor (arrows) has no associated calcifications.

Analysis

Form: circumscribed, highly lobulated
Contour: partially unsharp, no halo sign
Density: low density radiopaque
Size: approximately 1 × 1 cm

Comment

Although this circumscribed tumor has low density, the contours are unsharp, which raises the suspicion of malignancy. This suspicion is strengthened by the fact that this tumor has developed within a short time in an 80-year-old woman. Mucinous and papillary carcinomas may have low density at mammography.

Conclusion

Any circumscribed radiopaque tumor with unsharp borders and no demonstrable halo sign should lead to the suspicion of malignancy, regardless of the density.

Histology

Mucinous carcinoma. No lymph node metastases.

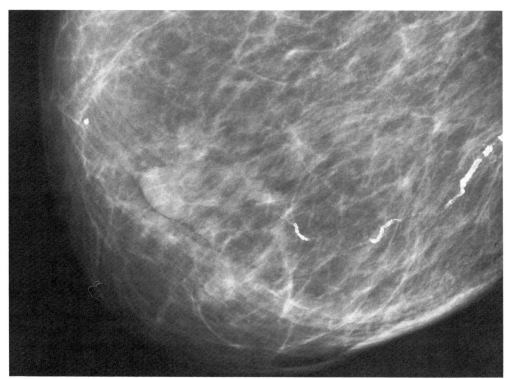

A

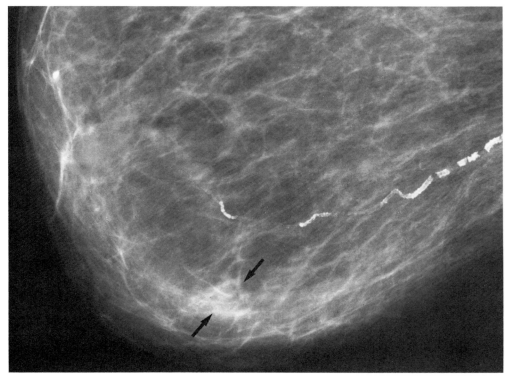

B

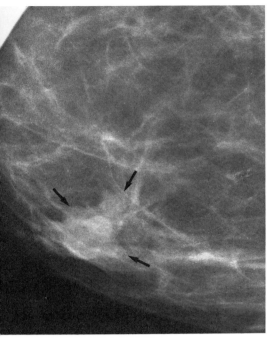

28 C

29

Age 74. The patient observed a slowly growing lump in the right breast over the past year.

Physical Examination

The palpable tumor in the right breast is clinically malignant.

Mammography

Fig. 29: Right breast, cranio-caudal view. A circumscribed tumor is seen 5 cm from the nipple in the central portion of the breast. There are no associated calcifications.

Analysis

Form: circumscribed, round, partially lobulated
Contour: ill-defined, spiculated
Density: high density radiopaque
Size: 2 × 2 cm

Conclusion

Mammographically malignant tumor.

Histology

Well differentiated ductal carcinoma. No lymph node metastases.

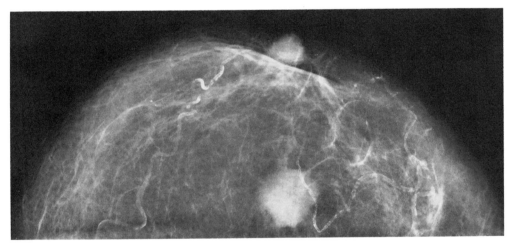

29

30

40-year-old asymptomatic woman. First screening study.

Physical Examination

No palpable tumor.

Mammography

Fig. 30 A: Right breast, cranio-caudal projection. A circumscribed tumor is located in the medial half of the breast. No associated calcifications.
Fig. 30 B & C: Microfocus magnification mammography in the cranio-caudal and latero-medial projections.
Fig. 30 D: Specimen radiograph with magnification.

Analysis

Form: circumscribed, oval
Contour: sharply outlined, no definite halo sign
Density: low density radiopaque
Size: 1 × 1 cm

Comment

Overlying parenchyma partially obscures the sharp borders of the tumor.

Conclusion

Mammographically benign tumor.

Histology

Fibroadenoma.

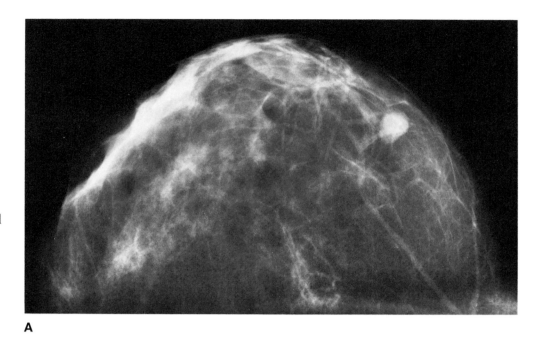

A

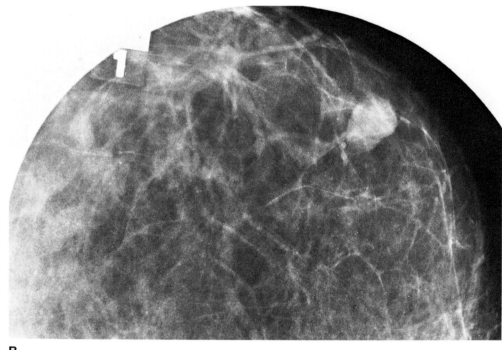

B

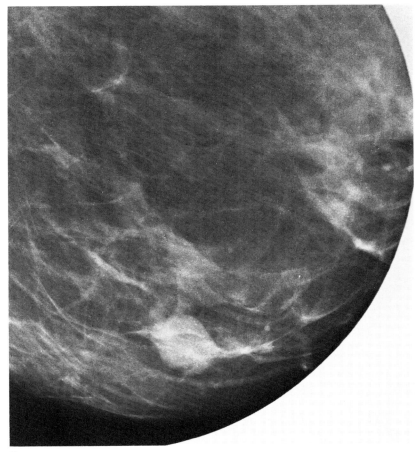

C

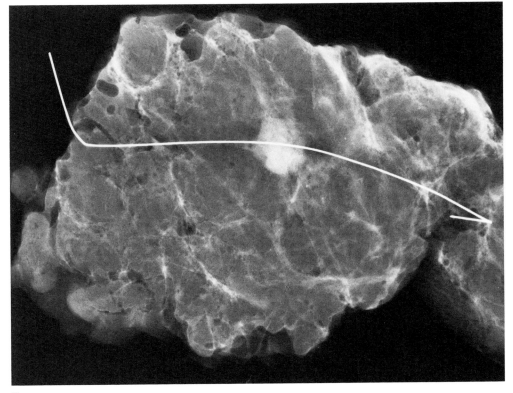

D

31

Fig. 31 A & B: Right breast, medio-lateral oblique and cranio-caudal projections. There is a solitary tumor in the upper outer quadrant. No associated calcifications.

Analysis

Form: circumscribed, oval
Contour: sharp
Density: low density radiopaque; a vein and parenchymal structures can be seen superimposed over the tumor
Size: 2 × 3 cm
Location: intra- and subdermal, protruding from the skin surface

Conclusion

Mammographically benign tumor. Clinical examination reveals a typical atheroma (sebaceous cyst).

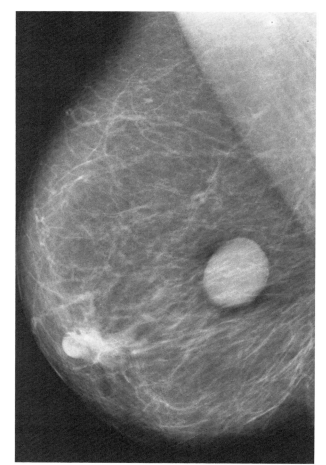

A

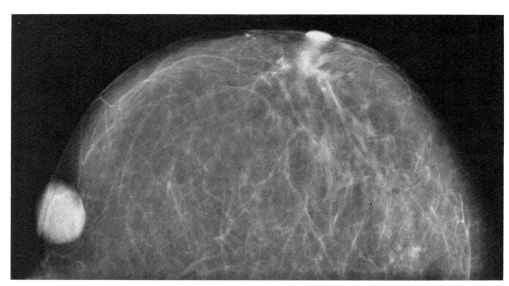

B

32

65-year-old woman, discovered a hard lump in the right breast one week earlier.

Physical Examination

6 × 6 cm freely movable tumor, hard at palpation. No skin changes.

Mammography

Fig. 32 A & B: Right breast, detailed views of the medio-lateral oblique and cranio-caudal projections show a circumscribed tumor with no associated calcifications.

Analysis

Form: circumscribed, lobulated
Contour: irregular, no halo sign
Density: low density radiopaque; structural elements can be seen through the tumor
Size: 5 × 5 cm

Conclusion

Though this circumscribed tumor is of low density, it is not sharply outlined and there is no halo sign. This should caution the reader: there are two malignant lesions that fit these criteria — mucinous and papillary carcinoma.

Histology

Mucinous carcinoma. No axillary metastases.

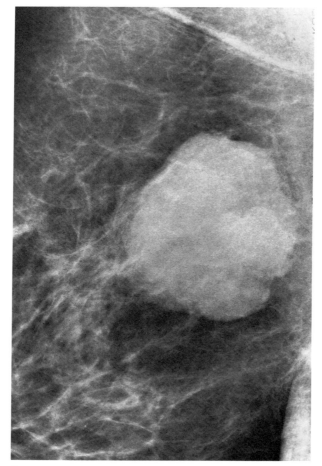

A

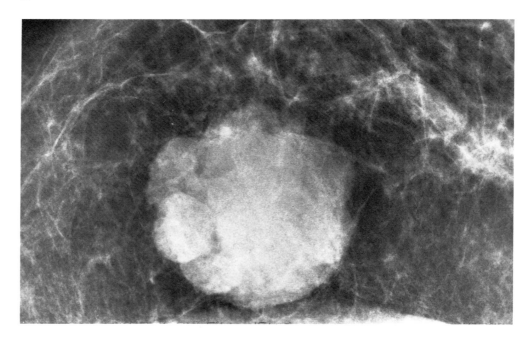

33

Asymptomatic 65-year-old woman. First screening study.

Physical Examination

No palpable tumor.

Mammography

Fig. 33 A & B: Left breast, medio-lateral oblique and cranio-caudal projections. A solitary tumor is seen in the upper outer quadrant. No associated calcifications.
Fig. 33 C & D: Microfocus magnification views in the medio-lateral oblique and cranio-caudal projections.

Analysis:

Form: circumscribed, oval
Contour: partly unsharp; an obvious comet tail is seen extending from the tumor in an anterior and caudal direction in A.
Density: high density radiopaque

Conclusion

Mammographically malignant tumor.
Fig. 33 E: Latero-medial view with biopsy localization plate.
Fig. 33 F: The hook localizes the tumor for biopsy.

Histology

Well differentiated ductal carcinoma, 7 × 6 mm. No axillary lymph node metastases.

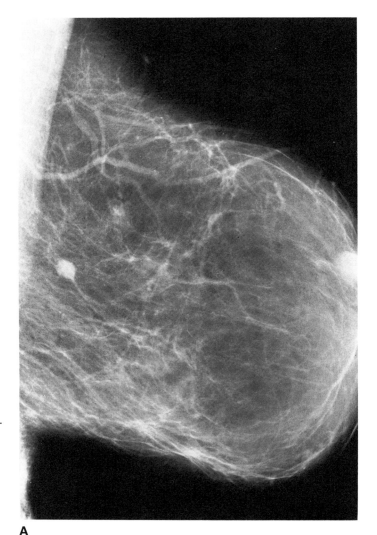

A

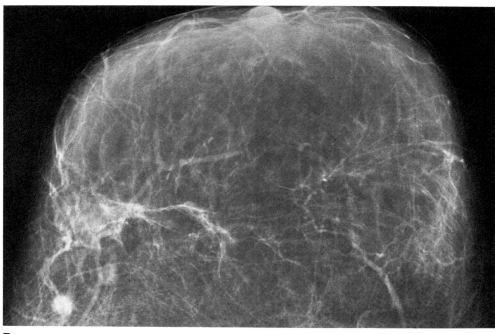

B

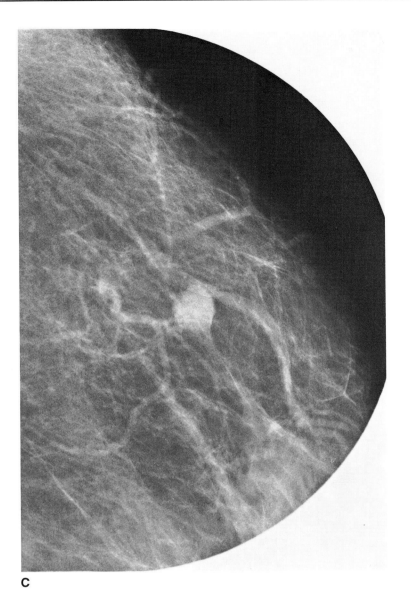

C

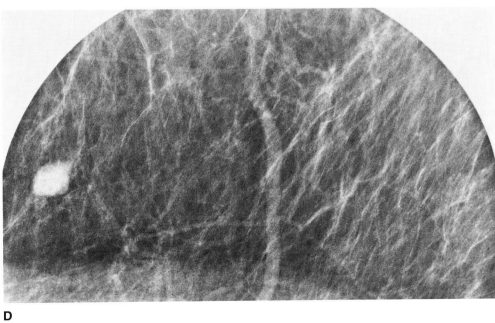

D

Fig. 33 E and F ▷

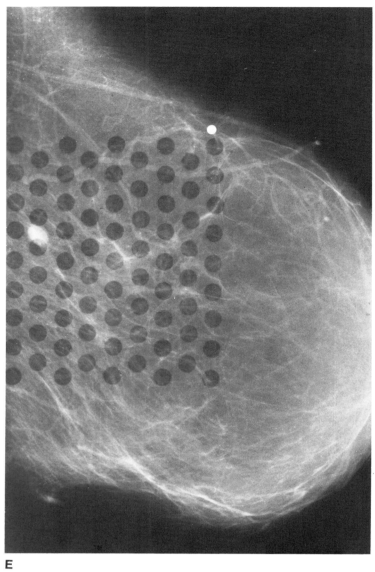

E

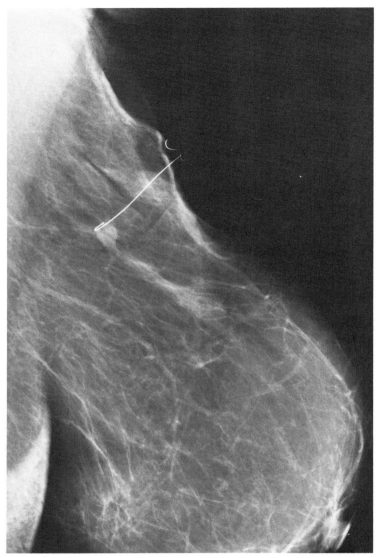

F

34

Asymptomatic 51-year-old woman. First screening study.

Physical Examination

Left upper outer quadrant contains a firm tumor mass. No skin changes.

Mammography

Fig. 34 A & B: Left breast, medio-lateral oblique and cranio-caudal projections. Numerous circumscribed tumors of varying size are seen in the upper outer quadrant. No associated calcifications.

Analysis of the Tumors

Form: circumscribed, lobulated, oval
Contour: sharply outlined
Density: low density radiopaque
Sizes: ½ to 4 cm

Conclusion

A group of mammographically benign tumors.

Cytology

Benign epithelial cells.

Histology

Multiple fibroadenomas. No evidence of malignancy.

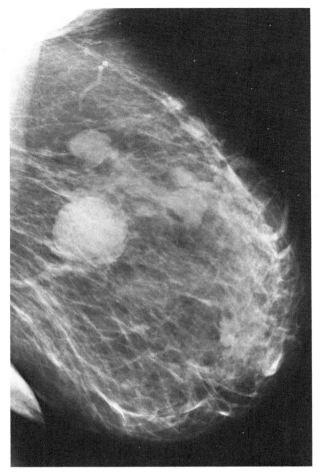

A

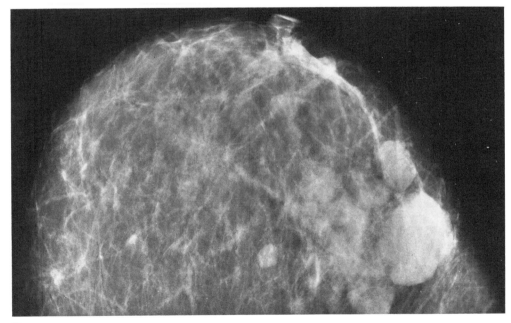

B

35

57-year-old asymptomatic woman, first screening study.

Mammography

Fig. 35 A: Left breast, detail of the medio-lateral oblique projection. No mammographic abnormality.
Fig. 35 B – D: Second screening examination *three years later*. Left breast, details of the medio-lateral oblique and cranio-caudal projections. Four cm from the nipple there is a 6 mm, lobulated, circumscribed tumor in the upper half of the breast.

Analysis

Form: circumscribed, lobulated
Contour: unsharp, no halo sign
Density: low density radiopaque
Size: 6 × 4 mm

Comment

De novo appearance of an unsharp, lobulated, circumscribed tumor in a 60-year-old woman leads to the suspicion of malignancy.

Histology

Noninfiltrating intraductal carcinoma, diameter 6 mm.

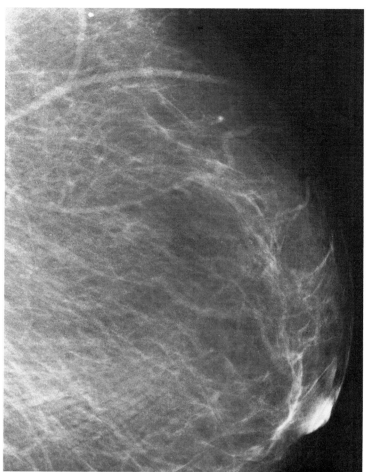

A

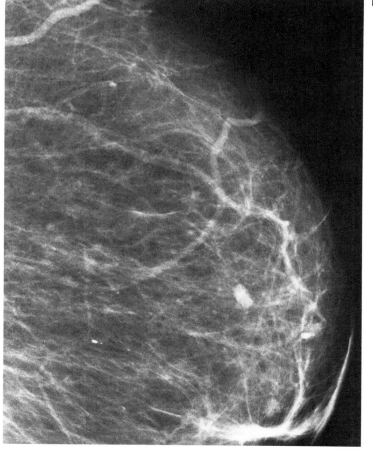

B

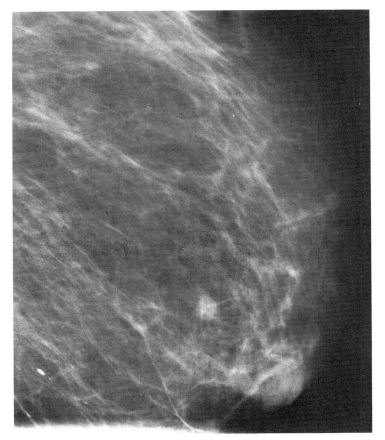

C

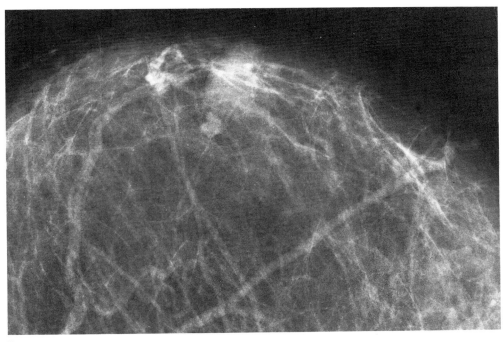

D

36

66-year-old asymptomatic woman. First screening study.

Mammography

Fig. 36 A: Right breast, medio-lateral oblique projection. Normal mammogram.

Two years later the patient presents with a two month history of a mass in the axillary portion of the right breast and a mass in the right iliac fossa.

Repeat Mammography

Fig. 36 B: Right breast, medio-lateral oblique projection. A tumor is seen high up in the axillary portion of the breast. No associated calcifications.

Analysis

Form: circumscribed, lobulated
Contour: partly sharply outlined, but there are also short spicules extending from the tumor periphery
Density: high density radiopaque
Size: 3 × 2½ cm

Conclusion

Mammographically malignant tumor. It has developed over less than two years, is highly dense, and has unsharp borders with short spicules.

Histology

Lymphoma (both in the breast and in the iliac fossa).

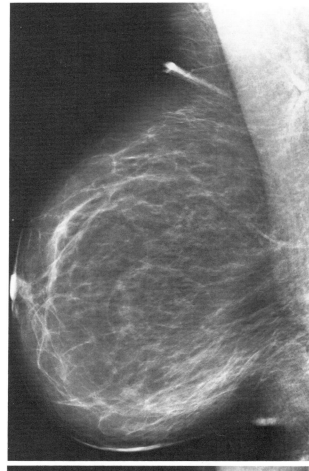

A

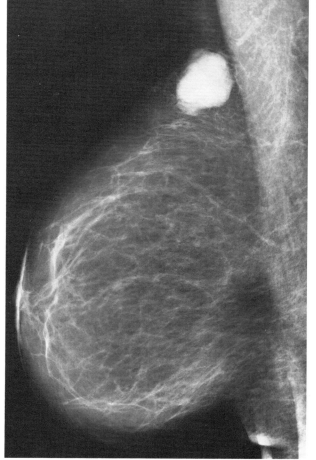

B

37

49-year-old woman with a 6 × 4 cm hard, centrally located, freely movable tumor in the left breast.

Physical Examination

Benign tumor.

Mammography

Fig. 37: Left breast, cranio-caudal projection. A large centrally located tumor with no associated calcifications.

Analysis

Form: circumscribed, lobulated
Contour: sharply outlined (part of the contour is obscured by the retroareolar fibrosis), no halo sign
Density: high
Size: 6 × 5 cm

Comment

A huge, sharply outlined, radiopaque tumor in a woman of menopausal age raises the suspicion of a cyst or cystosarcoma phylloides. Puncture provides differentiation.

Conclusion

Mammographically benign tumor.

Histology

Cystosarcoma phylloides.

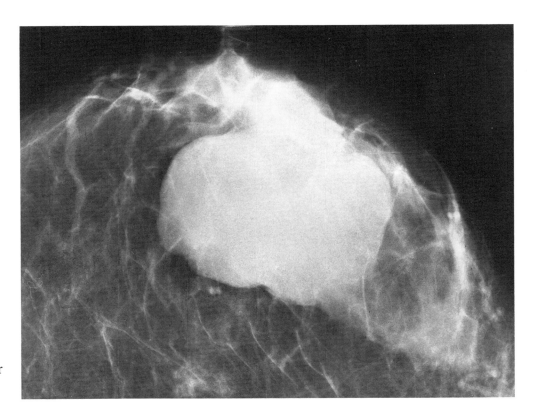

38

40-year-old woman, first noted a rapidly growing retroareolar tumor of the left breast four weeks earlier, associated with fever, pain, tenderness and periareolar erythema.

Physical Examination

Inspection: 7 × 6 cm area of periareolar erythema and extensive *peau d'orange.*
Palpation: Left breast heavier than right. Warm, tender, large retroareolar tumor. Enlarged axillary lymph nodes.
The patient is febrile.

Mammography

Fig. 38 A & B: Medio-lateral oblique and cranio-caudal projection. There is a large, 7 × 6 cm, dense retroareolar tumor with unsharp borders. It is associated with nipple retraction and skin thickening over the areola and lower portions of the breast.

Comment

A huge retroareolar abscess or an inflammatory carcinoma could both produce this clinical picture. However, an inflammatory cancer would result in an extensive reticular pattern over most of the breast on the mammogram through axillary lymphatic obstruction. Puncture gives further help in differentiation.

Puncture

60 ml pus.
Fig. 38 C: Mammography of the left breast after puncture and air insufflation: A small amount of air is seen in the much contracted abscess cavity (arrow).

Follow-up

The patient was placed on oral antibiotics and nine days later the abscess was incised and drained.
Repeat mammography in the cranio-caudal projection (Fig. 38 D) five weeks later shows only a slight degree of fibrosis and no underlying tumor.

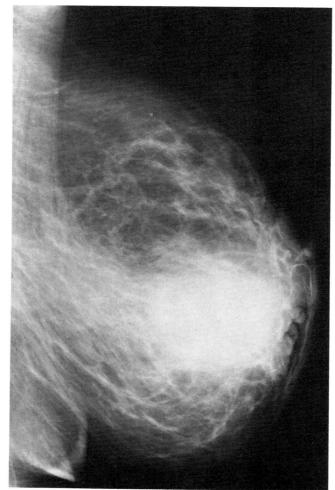

A

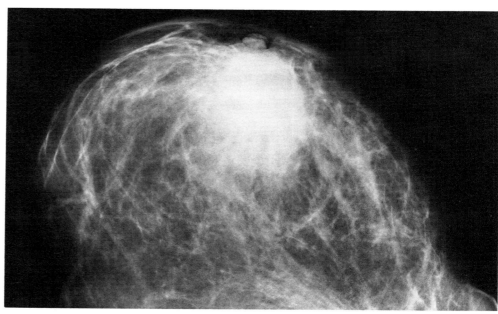

B

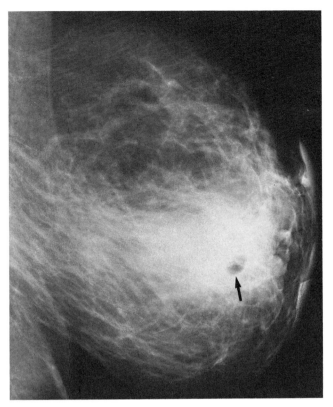

C

D

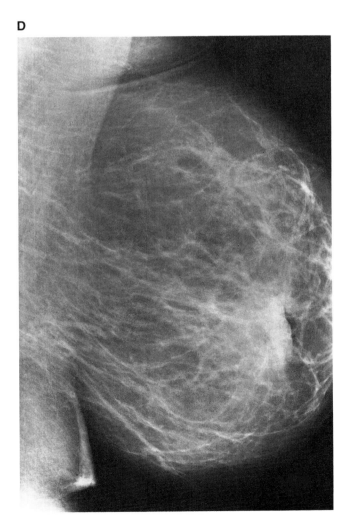

39

Age 36. The patient discovered a lump in her right breast 2 weeks earlier.

Physical Examination

2 cm freely movable tumor in the upper inner quadrant of the right breast. No skin changes.

Mammography

Fig. 39 A & B: Right breast, medio-lateral oblique and cranio-caudal projections. There is an oval-shaped tumor in the upper inner quadrant with no associated calcifications.

Analysis

Form: circumscribed, oval shaped
Contour: mostly ill-defined; there is a short segment of halo sign (arrows)
Density: low density radiopaque
Size: 3 × 2½ cm

Conclusion

The mostly ill-defined tumor margin leads to the suspicion of malignancy in spite of the short halo sign. Puncture is recommended.

Puncture

5 ml straw-coloured fluid aspirated.

Cytology

Inflammatory cells. No malignant cells. Abscess? Inflamed cyst?
Fig. 39 C & D: Pneumocystography. The inferior and anterior wall of the cyst is sharp, but the upper and posterior wall is irregular and thickened, best seen on the cranio-caudal projection (Fig. 39 D). Tumor in the cyst wall?

Histology

Medullary cancer in a 2 cm segment of the wall of a cyst.

Comment

This case demonstrates the diagnostic value of pneumocystography.

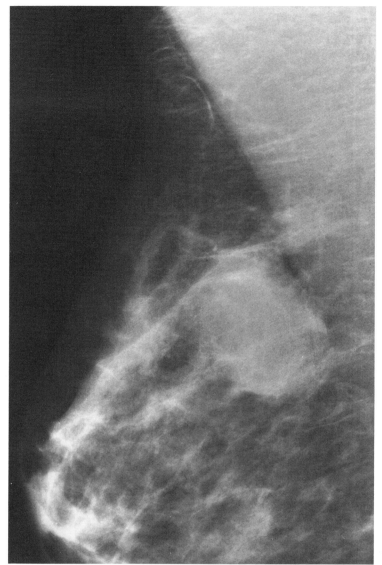

A

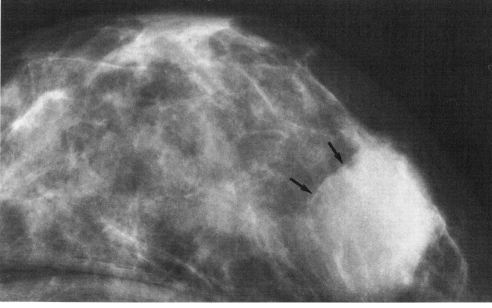

B

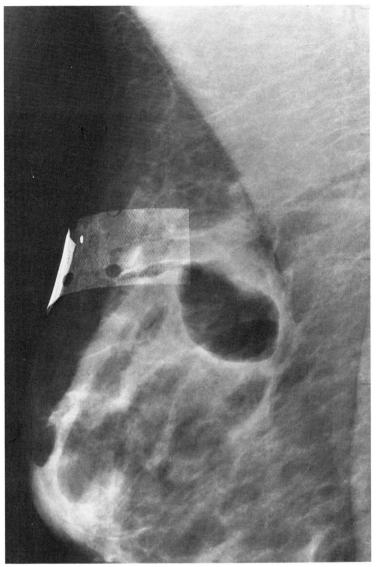

C

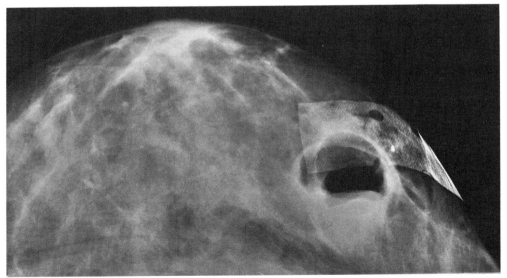

D

67

40

49-year-old woman with a one-and-a half year history of malignant melanoma. She now seeks medical attention for a mass in the right breast and in both axillas.

Physical Examination

There is a hard, freely movable lump in the lateral half of the right breast, 10 cm from the nipple, and large axillary lymph nodes.

Mammography

Fig. 40: Right breast, medio-lateral oblique projection shows two circumscribed tumors near the chest wall.

Analysis of the Larger Tumor

Form: circumscribed, lobulated
Contour: unsharp, spiculated
Density: high density radiopaque
Size: 4 cm

Conclusion

This is a mammographically malignant tumor.

Histology

Malignant melanoma metastases.

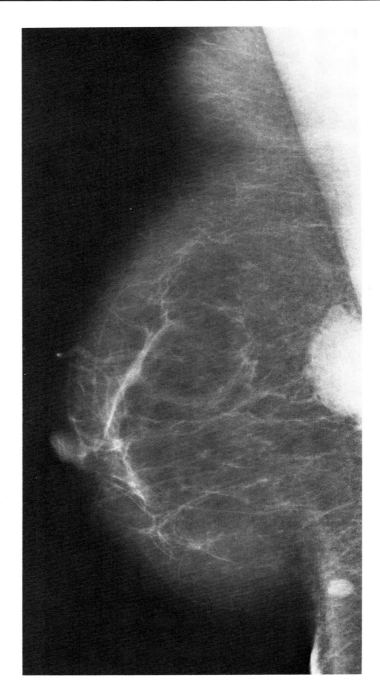

41

66-year-old woman referred for a self-detected lump in the upper outer quadrant of the right breast, clinically suspicious for malignancy.

Mammography

Fig. 41 A: Right breast, medio-lateral oblique projection. There is a circumscribed tumor 4 cm from the nipple, in the upper half of the breast. No associated calcifications.

Fig. 41 B: Enlargement of the coned-down compression view of the tumor.

Analysis

Form: circumscribed, circular
Contour: short spicules radiating from the tumor periphery
Density: high density radiopaque

Conclusion

Mammographically malignant tumor.

Histology

Partly ductal, partly papillary carcinoma. No lymph node metastases.

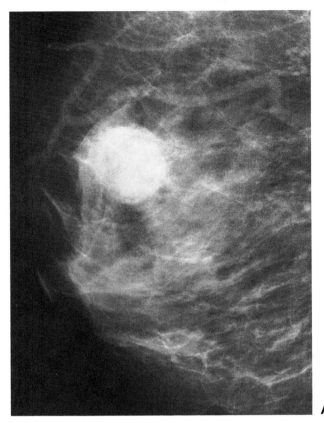

A

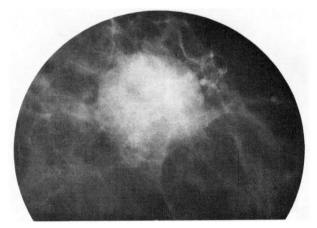

B

42

45-year-old woman detected a lump in her left breast one month earlier.

Physical Examination

10 cm tumor located centrally in the left breast. *Peau d'orange* over the lower half of the breast but no signs of inflammation.

Mammography

Fig. 42 A & B: Left breast, medio-lateral oblique and cranio-caudal projections. A large, circumscribed, oval tumor fills in the central portion of the breast. No associated calcifications. The pectoral muscle appears to be infiltrated. There is a pathologically enlarged lymph node in the axilla. No skin thickening, no reticular pattern on the mammogram, i.e., no mammographic signs of lymphedema.

Analysis

Form: circumscribed, oval
Contour: unsharp, no halo sign
Density: high density radiopaque
Size: 10 × 10 cm

Comment

Both malignancy and abscess are suggested by the high density, unsharp contour and infiltration of the pectoral muscle. However, a malignant tumor of this size with associated enlarged axillary lymph nodes and *peau d'orange* would be expected to cause lymphedema (skin thickening and a reticular pattern over much of the breast). Puncture is necessary for differential diagnosis.

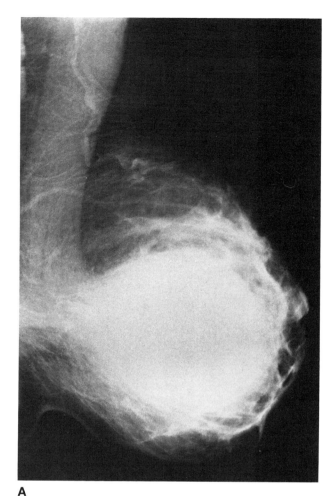

A

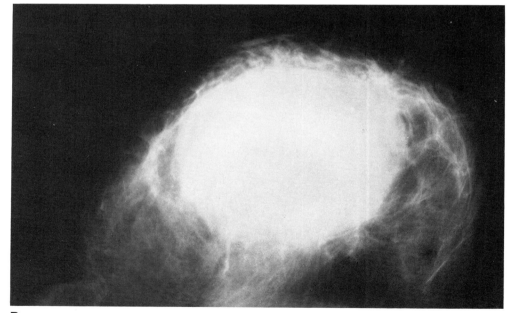

B

Fig. 42 C & D: Left breast, medio-lateral oblique and cranio-caudal projections after *puncture,* removal of 80 ml pus, and insufflation of air.

Conclusion

Abscess with a thick, irregular wall.

Histology

Abscess, no evidence of malignancy.

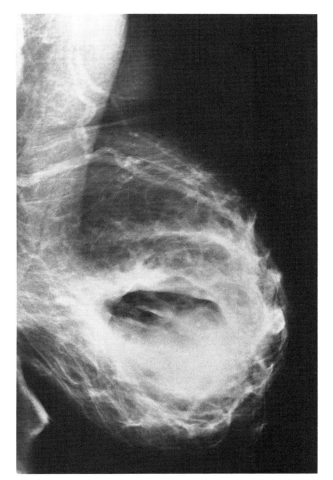

C

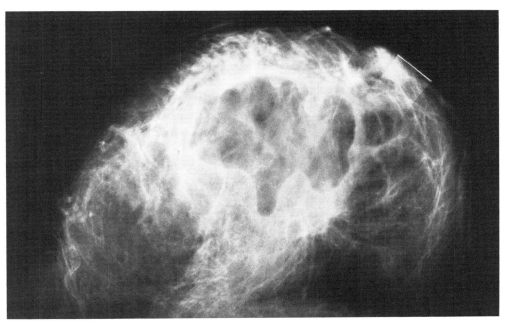

D

43

Asymptomatic woman, age 55. First screening study.

Physical Examination

No abnormalities in the breasts. Enlarged axillary lymph nodes bilaterally

Mammography

Fig. 43 A: Left breast, medio-lateral oblique projection. Normal breast. Enlarged, dense axillary lymph nodes.

Comment

When the axillary lymph nodes are enlarged and breast disease can be ruled out with certainty by physical examination and mammography, the following diagnoses should be considered: lymphoma, leukemia and rheumatoid arthritis.

Magnification Immersion Radiography of the Left Hand

Radiographic changes in the soft tissues and bone, typical of rheumatoid arthritis (Fig. 43 B).

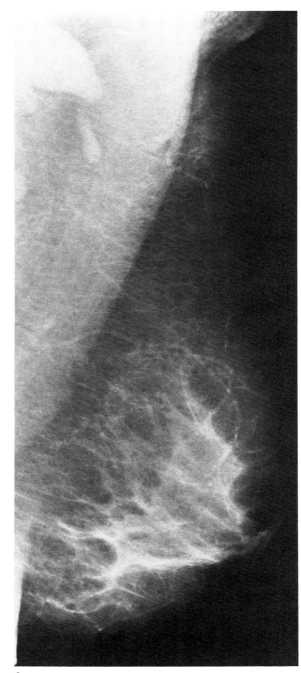

A

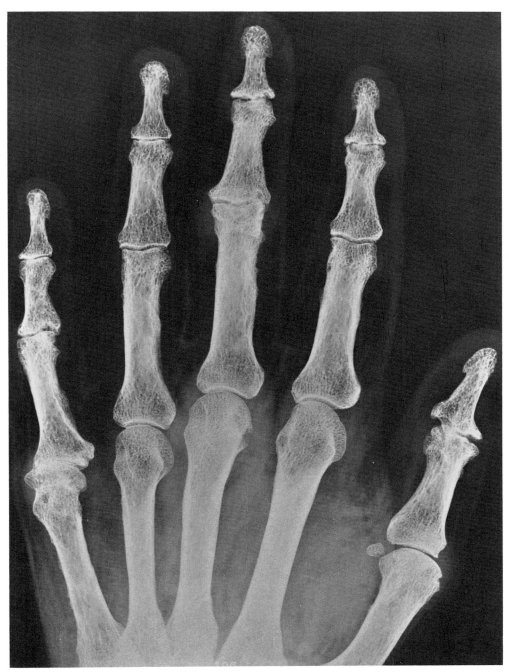

B

44

82-year-old woman noticed a lump in her left breast.

Physical Examination

Freely movable tumor below the nipple, clinically benign.

Mammography

Fig. 44 A: Left breast, medio-lateral oblique projection, detailed view of the lower half of the breast.
Fig. 44 B: Left breast, cranio-caudal projection, detailed view.
Fig. 44 C & D: Left breast, micro-focus magnification views in the medio-lateral oblique and cranio-caudal projections.
There is a solitary tumor with no associated calcifications 5 cm from the sharply outlined nipple.

Analysis

Form: circumscribed, lobulated
Contour: unsharp, no halo sign; compare with the nipple, which is sharply outlined
Density: low density radiopaque
Size: 1 × 1 cm

Conclusion

The unsharp borders and absence of a halo sign make this circumscribed tumor, newly occuring in an 82-year-old woman, suggest a malignancy.

Histology

Mucinous carcinoma. No axillary metastases.

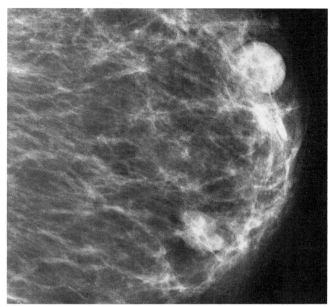

A

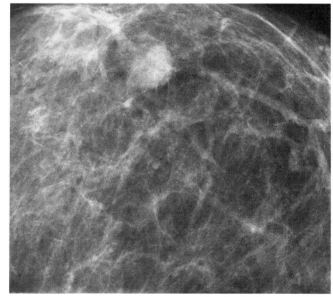

B

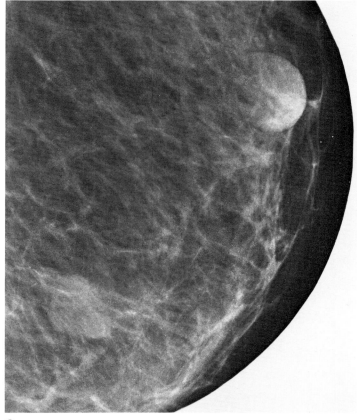

C

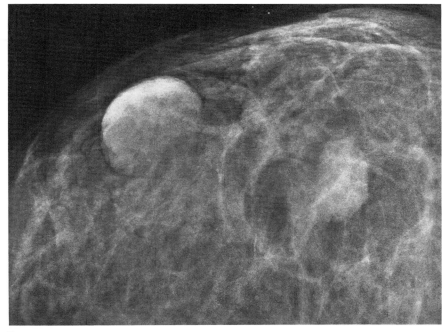

D

45

Fig. 45 A & B: Mammographic picture of pathologically enlarged axillary lymph nodes in a 68-year-old woman with chronic lymphatic leukemia.

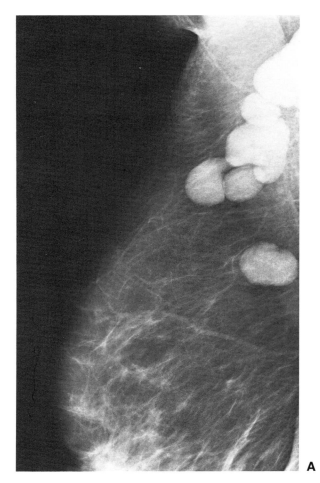

A

B

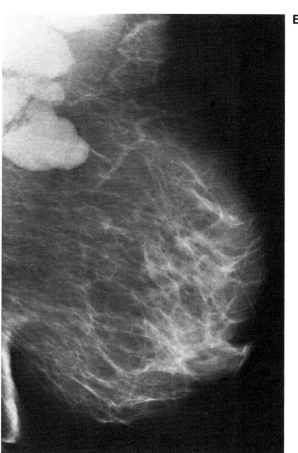

46

63-year-old woman, asymptomatic, second screening examination.

Physical Examination

No palpable tumor.

Mammography

Fig. 46 A: Right breast, medial portion of the cranio-caudal projection. A solitary tumor is seen 6 cm from the nipple. No associated calcifications.

Analysis

Form: circumscribed, lobulated
Contour: the medial border is sharply outlined with a halo sign
Density: low density radiopaque
Size: 2 × 1½ cm

Conclusion

Mammographically benign tumor which has developed since the first screening examination three years earlier.

Fine Needle Biopsy

Fig. 46 B: Detailed view of the lesion following puncture. Typical mammographic appearance of a hematoma, which hides the tumor completely.

Cytology

Benign epithelial cells.
Fig. 46 C: Two weeks later, preoperative localization. The resolving hematoma still obscures the tumor.

Histology

Benign intraductal papilloma and cystic hyperplasia.

Comment

As this case clearly demonstrates, a hematoma caused by fine needle puncture can completely obscure a breast tumor, making the mammographic diagnosis impossible. For this reason fine needle puncture should never precede mammography (ref. 54).

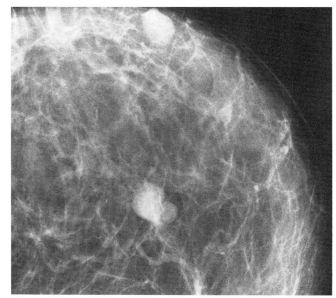

A

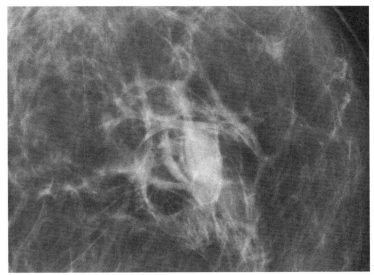

B

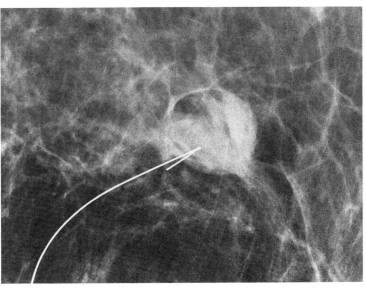

C

47

47-year-old woman, asymptomatic. First screening study.

Physical Examination

No palpable tumor.

Mammography

Fig. 47 A: Right breast, medio-lateral oblique projection. A tumor is seen in the upper half of the breast, 6 cm from the nipple.
Fig. 47 B: Enlarged view of the tumor.

Analysis

Form: circumscribed, oval, lobulated
Contour: partly unsharp, no halo sign
Density: radiolucent and radiopaque combined (central radiolucency)
Size: approx. 1 cm

Conclusion

The mixed density is the crucial factor determining the benign nature of this tumor. Further differential diagnosis follows that described in the Conclusion of Case 9.
The radiolucent part corresponds to the hilus of this *intramammary lymph node.*

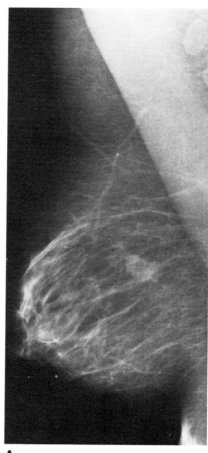

A

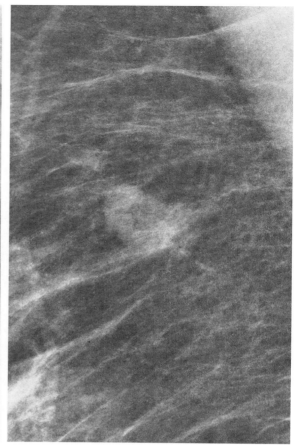

B

48

29-year-old woman, first detected a lump in the upper lateral quadrant of the left breast two months earlier.

Physical Examination

An élongated, firm, movable, nodular tumor extending from the nipple to the upper outer quadrant, clinically benign.

Mammography

Fig. 48 A & B: Left breast, cranio-caudal projection, contact and magnification views of the lateral half of the breast. A 10 cm long, multinodular tumor resembling a set of rosary beads extends laterally from the nipple. There are associated calcifications.

Analysis of the Tumor

Form: elongate, multinodular
Contour: smooth, undulating
Density: low density radiopaque
Distribution: fills in an entire lobe

Conclusion

The mammographic appearance is that of the dilated duct system of a single lobe.

Analysis of the Calcifications

Form: irregular
Density: the largest calcification appears hollow and the smaller calcifications are very dense
Contour: smooth, regular
Location: within the dilated ducts

Comment

Mammographically benign type calcifications, most likely papillomatosis (page 173).

Conclusion

The multiple intraductal calcifications, typical of papillomatosis, within an irregularly dilated duct system of a lobe in a young woman, suggest the diagnosis of juvenile papillomatosis (Swiss cheese disease).

Histology

Juvenile Papillomatosis.

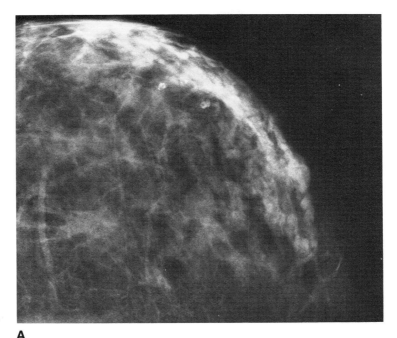

A

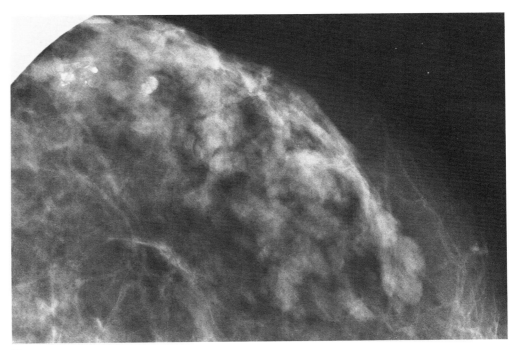

B

49

Fig. 49 A & B: Right breast, detailed views from the medio-lateral oblique and cranio-caudal projections. Solitary tumor, no associated calcifications.

Analysis

Form: circumscribed, oval
Contour: halo sign over much of the border
Density: low density radiopaque, details of parenchymal structure can be seen superimposed on the tumor

Conclusion

Mammographically benign tumor. At puncture the tumor was solid.

Cytology

Benign epithelial cells.

Histology

Fibroadenoma.

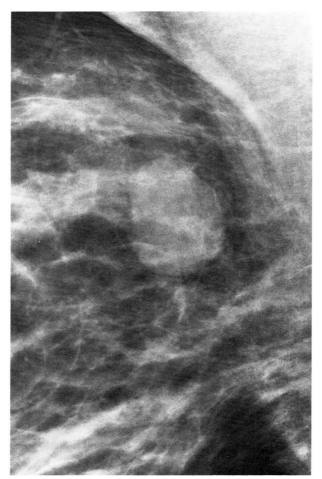

A

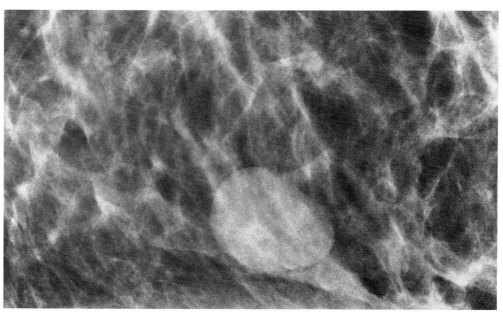

B

50

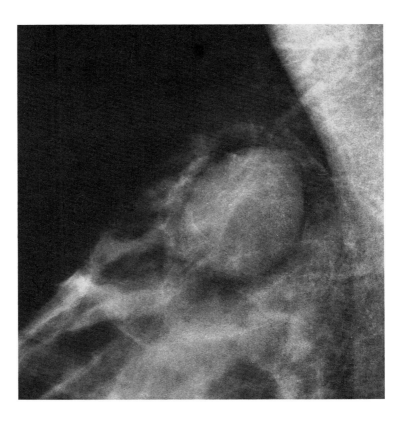

Fig. 50: Right breast, detail from the medio-lateral oblique projection. Solitary tumor, no calcification.

Analysis

Form: circumscribed, oval
Contour: sharply outlined, definite halo sign along the posterior border
Density: low density radiopaque; vein and parenchymal elements can be seen superimposed on the tumor
Size: 4 × 3 cm

Conclusion

All mammographic signs indicate a benign tumor.

Histology

Fibroadenoma.

51

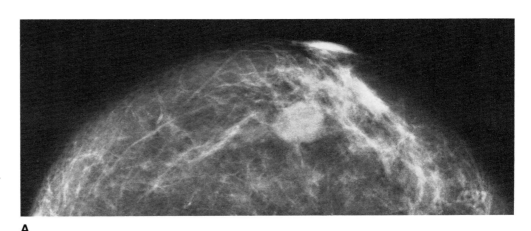

A

Fig. 51 A: Right breast, cranio-caudal projection. A 2 cm solitary tumor in the central portion of the breast with no associated calcifications.
Fig. 51 B: Coned-down enlarged view of the tumor, cranio-caudal projection.

Analysis

Form: circumscribed, oval
Contour: unsharp, poorly defined; no definite halo sign demonstrated even on the coned-down compression view
Density: low density radiopaque; equal to the parenchyma
Size: 15 × 12 mm

Conclusion

The poorly defined borders of the tumor raise the suspicion of malignancy, making biopsy mandatory.

Histology

Fibroadenoma. No evidence of malignancy.

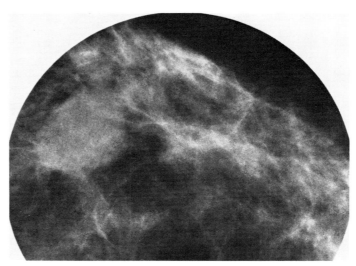

B

52

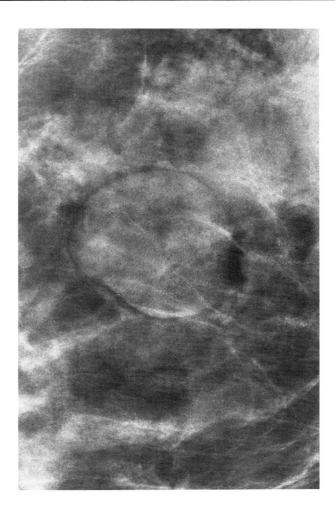

Fig. 52: Enlargement from the medio-lateral oblique projection.

Analysis

Form: circumscribed, oval
Contour: sharply outlined, halo sign surrounding the entire tumor
Density: low density radiopaque, equal to parenchyma; parenchymal elements are clearly seen overlying the tumor

Conclusion

Mammographically benign tumor, cyst.

Comment

Extraordinarily prominent halo sign. Puncture: 7 ml straw-coloured fluid. No intracystic tumor on pneumocystography.

53

Age 71, palpable tumor in the lateral half of the left breast, clinically benign.

Mammography

Fig. 53 A: Left breast, detailed view of the medio-lateral oblique projection. There is a solitary tumor in the breast with no associated calcifications.

Analysis

Form: circumscribed, oval
Contour: sharply outlined, extensive halo sign along the superior border
Density: low density radiopaque

Conclusion

Mammographically benign tumor, with a cyst as the most likely diagnosis. Puncture and pneumocystography are recommended to confirm the diagnosis and provide therapy.
Fig. 53 B: Pneumocystogram. The cyst has been emptied and filled with air. There is no intracystic tumor (bubbles are seen in the remaining cyst fluid).

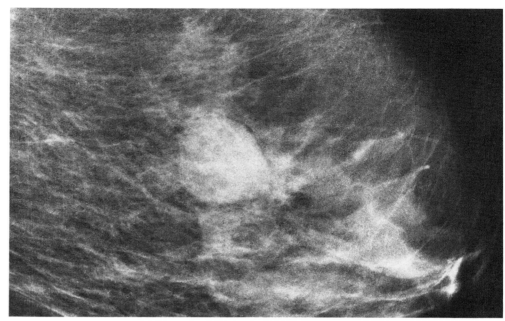

A

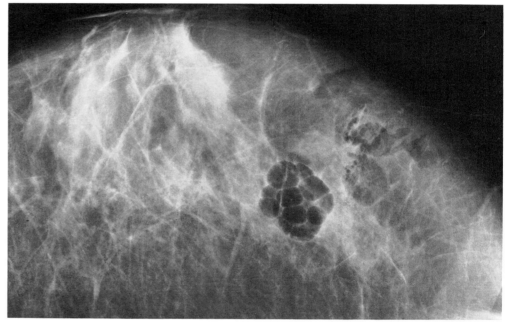

B

54

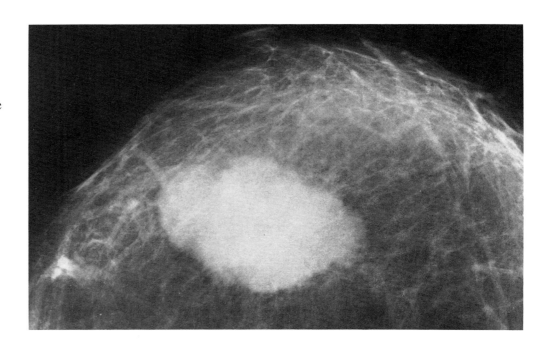

Fig. 54: Detailed mammogram in the cranio-caudal projection. 6 × 4 cm lobulated tumor without associated calcifications.

Analysis

Form: circumscribed, oval-shaped, lobulated
Contour: not sharply outlined, many short spicules seen on the entire contour
Density: high density radiopaque
Size: 6 × 4 cm

Conclusion

Mammographically typical malignant tumor.

Histology

Carcinoma.

55

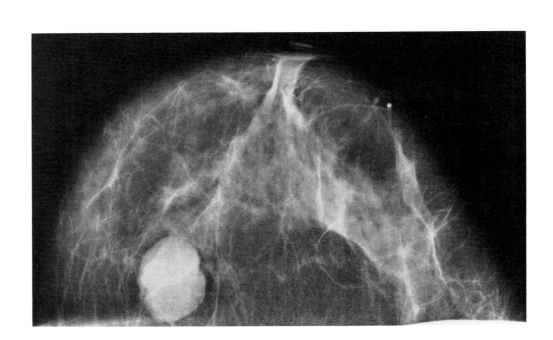

Fig. 55: Left breast, cranio-caudal projection. There is a tumor in the medial half of the breast, near the chest wall.

Analysis

Form: circumscribed, lobulated
Contour: sharply defined
Density: low density radiopaque
Size: 3½ × 2½ cm

Conclusion

Mammographically benign tumor.

Histology

Fibroadenoma.

56

Fig. 56 A: Right breast, detailed view of the cranio-caudal projection. A solitary tumor is seen without associated calcifications.

Analysis

Form: circumscribed, oval
Contour: lobulated, smooth; extensive halo sign
Density: low density radiopaque

Conclusion

Mammographically benign tumor. The extensive halo sign suggests a cyst.
Fig. 56 B: Pneumocystogram. Simple cyst; no intracystic tumor.

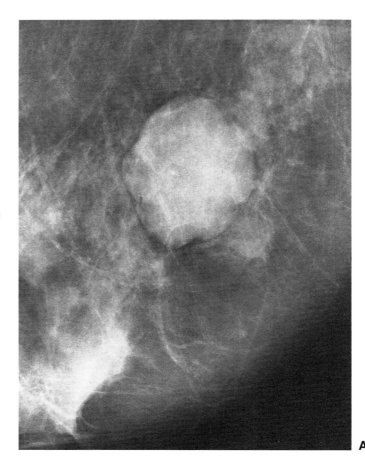

A

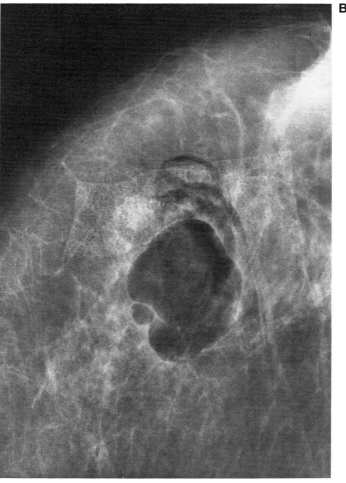

B

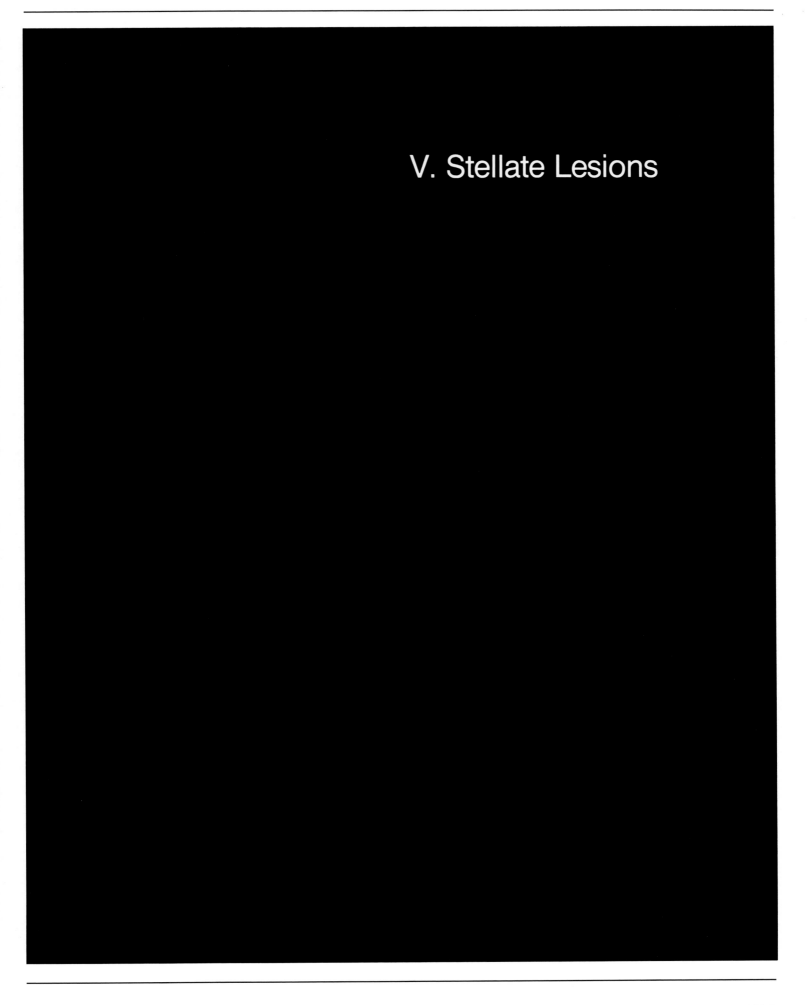

V. Stellate Lesions

Most breast carcinomas have the mammographic appearance of a stellate lesion, i. e. a radiating structure with ill-defined borders. Their *perception* may be difficult, especially when they are small.

Although mammographic differentiation of breast carcinoma from other stellate lesions can be highly accurate, definitive diagnosis can be made only by histology.

When *analyzing stellate lesions* the following radiologic signs should be considered:

Tumor center

a) Is it a distinct mass?

b) Instead of a solid, distinct mass are there oval or circular radiolucent areas at the center of the radiating structure?

Note: Coned-down compression views are of great value in evaluating the tumor center.

Radiating structure consisting of spicules. Two basic patterns:

a) Sharp, dense, fine lines of variable length radiating in all directions are typical of scirrhous carcinoma. The larger the central tumor mass the longer the spicules (Fig. XIV) (cases 57, 58, 59, 60, 65).

b) Many very fine spicules may be bunched together like a broom or a sheaf of wheat. Both these individual spicules and the radiating structures they form are of lower density than the corresponding structures in scirrhous carcinoma. This type of radiating structure is characteristic of sclerosing duct hyperplasia (Fig. XV) (cases 61, 62, 63, 64, 66, 67), and is occasionally seen in traumatic fat necrosis as well (case 68).

In addition, localized skin thickening and retraction over the lesion should be searched for. It is often present in scirrhous carcinoma, particularly in large and superficial lesions (case 60). It may be present in traumatic fat necrosis, especially postoperatively (cases 68, 69).

Sclerosing duct hyperplasia is never associated with skin thickening or retraction, no matter how large or superficial the lesion may be (cases 62, 64, 66, 67).

The analysis of the stellate lesions, according to the above mentioned signs, leads to a choice among the following diagnoses:

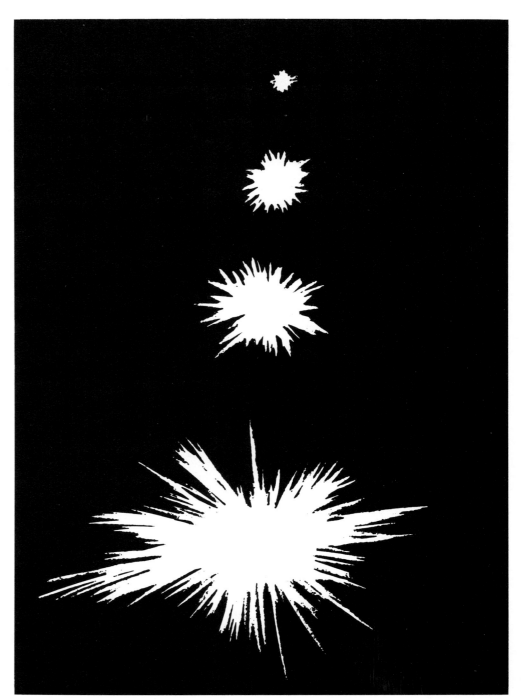

Fig. XIV: Diagrammatic illustration of scirrhous carcinoma: the larger the central tumor mass the longer the spicules.

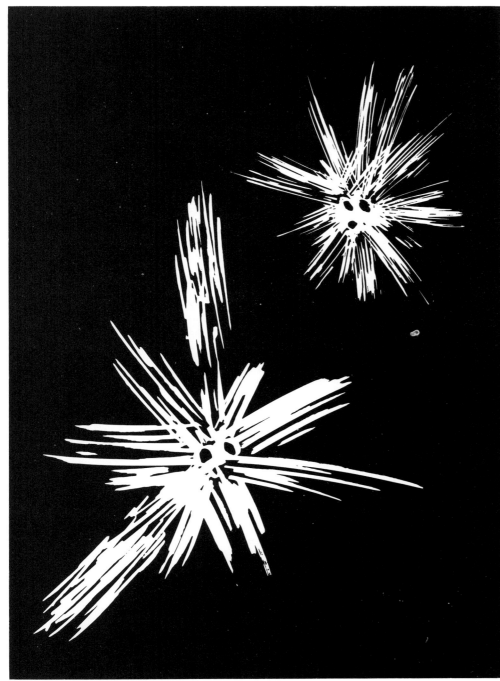

Fig. XV: Illustration of the mammographic appearance of sclerosing duct hyperplasia.

1) scirrhous carcinoma (infiltrating duct carcinoma)
2) small scirrhous carcinoma, early stage ("baby scirrhous")
3) sclerosing duct hyperplasia
4) traumatic fat necrosis
5) hyalinized fibroadenoma

Scirrhous carcinoma (infiltrating duct carcinoma) has the following mammographic characteristics (Fig. XIV) (cases 57, 58, 59, 60, 65, 70, 71, 72, 73, 85):
a) Distinct central tumor mass from which dense spicules radiate in all directions.
b) Spicule length increases with tumor size.
c) Spicules that may reach the skin or muscle, causing retraction and localized skin thickening.
d) Associated malignant-type calcifications are common.

Small scirrhous carcinoma, early stage ("baby scirrhous") (cases 74, 75, 76, 77, 78, 79, 80). Histopathologically not a separate entity but the radiologic appearance can differ from that described in the first group:
a) The perception problem can be considerable.
b) The central tumor mass may be imperceptible; although small, it is almost always present.
c) Spicules may form only a lace-like, fine reticular structure which causes parenchymal distortion and/or asymmetry. These may be the only changes leading to detection.

Comment: Coned-down compression views may be essential to separate these lesions from the summation of parenchymal structures.

Radial scar (sclerosing duct hyperplasia). This benign, rarely palpable lesion may be mistakenly diagnosed as carcinoma. Mammographic screening has focused attention upon this lesion. A prevalence of 0.9 per 1000 examined women was observed in our screening material.

The frequent occurrence of this cancer-imitating lesion in mammography screening makes it an important practical problem. Furthermore, the exact nature of this lesion is a subject of considerable controversy among pathologists and it has been given nine different names over the past 15 years (3, 4, 14, 15, 18, 21, 23, 32, 41).

The radiologist can facilitate proper final diagnosis by alerting the surgeon and the pathologist to this lesion. The following mammographic characteristics help to differentiate sclerosing duct hyperplasia from carcinoma even though biopsy is mandatory (cases 61, 62, 63, 64, 66, 67, 81, 82, 83) (Fig. XV).

a) The same lesion varies in appearance from one projection to the other. Each view gives a somewhat different picture.

b) There is no solid, dense, central tumor mass of a size corresponding to the length of the spicules. Instead, there are translucent, oval or circular areas at the center of the radiating structure which give it a striking appearance.

c) Spicules differ from those of scirrhous carcinoma. The longest are very thin and very long. Closer to the center of the lesion they may become much more numerous and are clumped together in thick aggregates.

d) There frequently appear to be radiolucent linear structures parallel to some of the spicules. These radiolucencies can dominate the radiographic picture (cases 61, 64, 81).

e) There is never skin thickening nor retraction over the lesion.

f) There is a striking difference between the distinct mammographic findings and the nearly complete absence of a palpable lesion, no matter how large or superficial it may be.

Traumatic fat necrosis. Fat necrosis following trauma, including surgery, can result in at least two basic types of radiologic images: a circumscribed lesion (oil cyst) and a stellate lesion. Calcification may be associated with either of them (Chapter VI). A complete history is essential for diagnosis. The presence of ecchymosis is useful. Characteristic mammographic appearance, when the traumatic fat necrosis results in a stellate lesion, is as follows (cases 66, 68, 84):

a) Center of the lesion: no distinct mass, instead translucent areas are within a loose, reticular structure. The older the lesion the less solid the center (cases 68, 84).

b) Radiating structure: varies with the projection, particularly in coned-down compression views. Spicules are fine and of low density.

c) Localized skin thickening and retraction may be present (cases 68, 69, 84).

Hyalinized fibroadenoma with fibrosis. Myxoid degeneration of a fibroadenoma may rarely result in retraction of the surrounding tissue which simulates a lesion with radiating structure (25). This pattern changes with each projection. It can be accompanied by the typical coarse calcification of fibroadenomas.

Strategy

Although definitive diagnosis of stellate lesions requires histologic examination, the preoperative mammographic analysis is important, because it should influence the surgeon's approach to the patient. The only stellate lesion which may be followed conservatively is postoperative traumatic fat necrosis.

Key Case

57

This case is meant to demonstrate the characteristics of a typical malignant stellate tumor.

It is recommended that you refer to this case while analyzing other stellate lesions.

It is the presence of a central tumor mass with associated spicules that is typical of malignant stellate tumors. The spicules are dense and sharp, radiating from the tumor surface, usually not bunched together. When they extend to the skin or areolar region they cause retraction and local thickening. The bigger the tumor mass the longer the spicules (Fig. XIV).

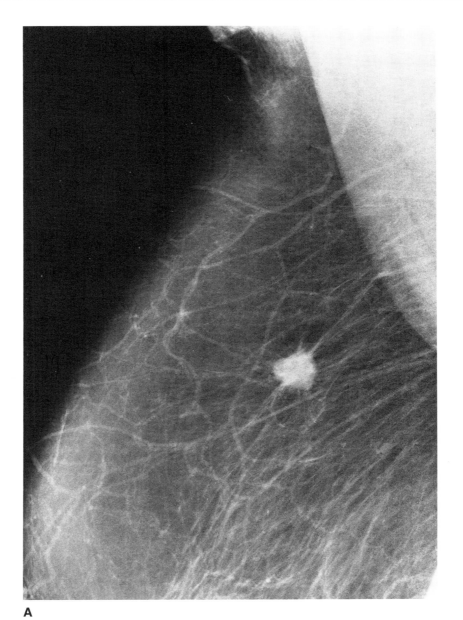

A

B

Practice in Analyzing Stellate Lesions

(Cases 58−85)

58

73-year-old asymptomatic woman. First screening study.

Physical Examination

No palpable tumor.

Mammography

Fig. 58 A: Right breast, medio-lateral oblique projection. A small tumor shadow is seen at coordinate A1.
Fig. 58 B: Right breast, cranio-caudal projection. The tumor is seen at coordinate A1. No associated calcifications.
Fig. 58 C: Magnification view, medio-lateral oblique projection.

Analysis

Form: small stellate tumor mass surrounded by spicules
Size: 4 × 4 mm

Conclusion

Mammographically malignant tumor.

Histology

Infiltrating ductal carcinoma, size 4 × 4 mm. No axillary metastases.
Fig. 58 D: Specimen photograph.

Fig. 58 D see Color Plate I, after p. 136.

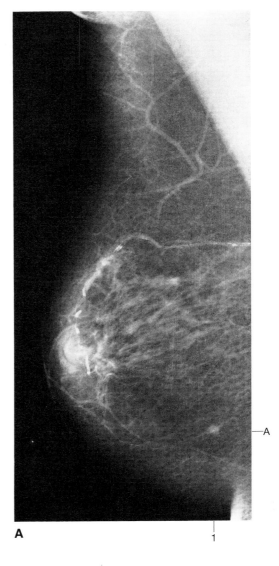

A   1

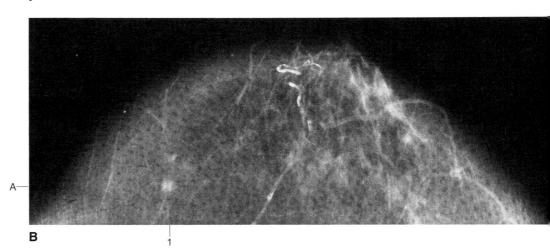

B   1

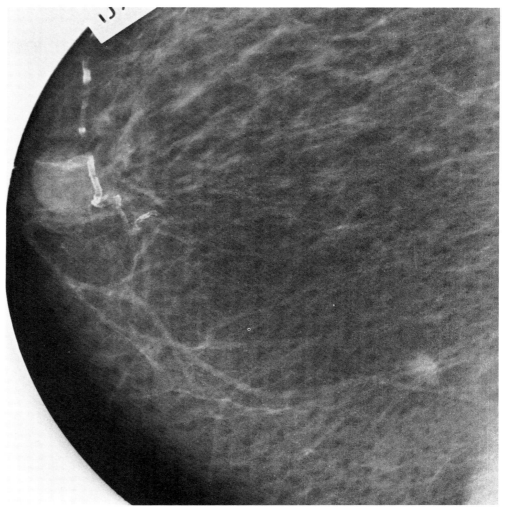

c

59

Age 63. First screening examination. Asymptomatic.

Physical Examination

No palpable tumor.

Mammography

Fig. 59 A: Left breast, medio-lateral oblique projection.
Fig. 59 B: Magnification view in the medio-lateral oblique projection.
Fig. 59 C: Left breast, cranio-caudal projection. A stellate tumor is seen in the upper inner quadrant, 7 cm from the nipple. No associated calcifications.

Conclusion

This tumor has the typical mammographic appearance of a malignant stellate breast tumor: solid center, radiating spicules.

Histology

Invasive ductal carcinoma. Maximum diameter 7 mm. No lymph node metastases.

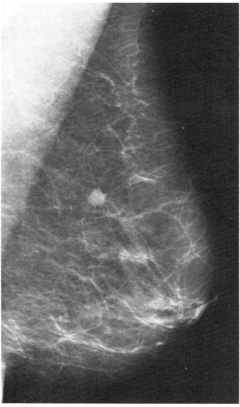

A

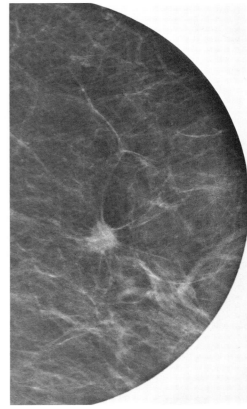

B

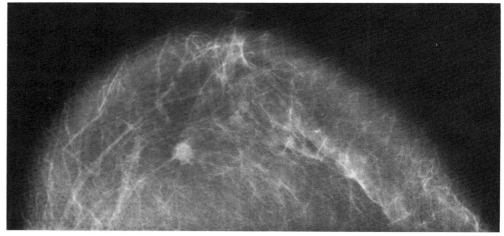

C

60

Age 89, one year history of a slowly growing tumor in the right breast.

Physical Examination

A large, obviously malignant tumor in the right breast.

Mammography

Fig. 60 A & B: Right breast, medio-lateral oblique and cranio-caudal projections. Centrally located, large (5 cm diameter) stellate tumor. The nipple and areola are retracted. The skin is thickened and retracted over the lower and outer portions of the breast.

Comment

An illustrative example of an advanced stellate malignant breast tumor with a large central tumor mass and radiating spicules which retract the areola and skin.

Histology

Infiltrating ductal carcinoma. The tumor infiltrates the lymph vessels.

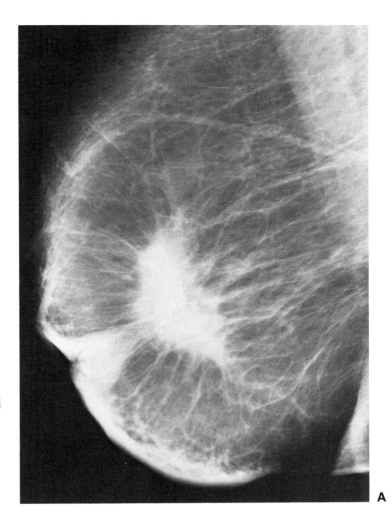

A

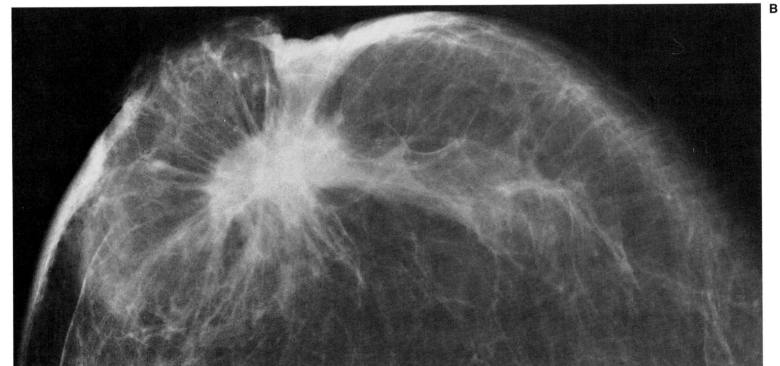

B

61

61-year-old woman, asymptomatic.
First screening study.

Physical Examination

No palpable tumor.

Mammography

Fig. 61 A & B: Right (A) and left (B) breasts, medio-lateral oblique projections. Compare the lower halves of the right and left breasts. In the lower half of the right breast there is a stellate lesion centered at coordinate A1.

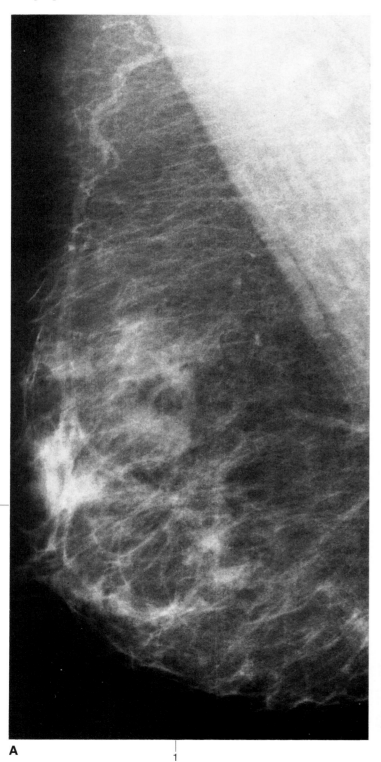

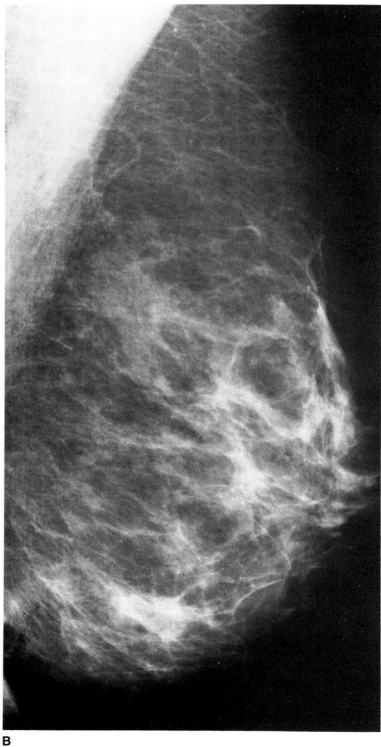

A   1   B

Fig. 61 D: Right breast, microfocus magnification view, medio-lateral oblique projection. Compare Fig. 61 A with Fig. 61 C & D. Observe how the lesion is different in each projection.

Analysis

Form: stellate; there is no central tumor mass; the magnification view in particular shows the small radiolucencies at the center of the lesion; the spicules are fine, extremely long, bunched together and extended to the nipple, which is not retracted
Size: large, fills in much of the lower outer breast quadrant

Conclusion

This mammographic appearance is typical of sclerosing duct hyperplasia.

Histology

Sclerosing duct hyperplasia (radial scar). No evidence of malignancy.

Comment

Any malignant tumor of this size will have a large, dense, homogeneous central tumor mass, which dominates the picture. In sclerosing duct hyperplasia the spicules form the lesion and, in contrast to carcinoma, there are numerous central translucencies.

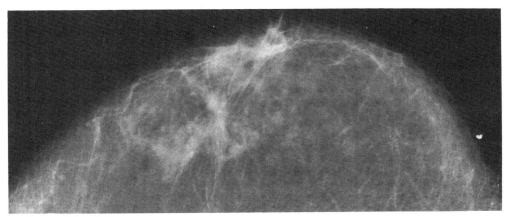

C

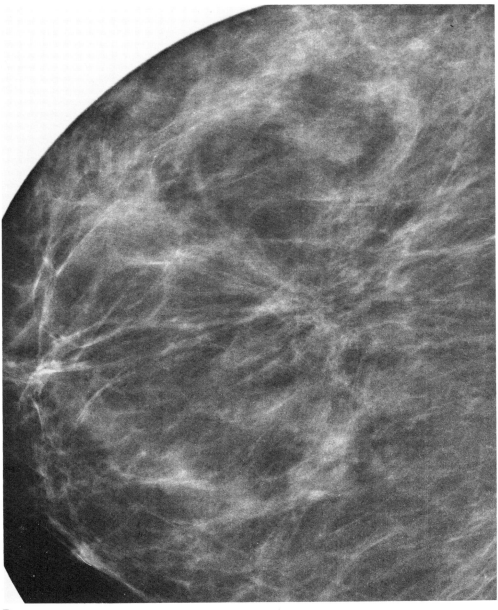

D

62

Age 63, asymptomatic. First screening study.

Physical Examination

No palpable tumor.

Mammography

Fig. 62 A & B: Medio-lateral and cranio-caudal projections. A large stellate lesion is centered 4 cm behind the nipple. Note the change in appearance of the lesion with changes in projection. The two benign-type periductal calcifications are not associated with the tumor.

Analysis

Stellate lesion, no solid central tumor mass. Radiolucencies are seen at the center in both projections, particularly in Fig. 62 A. Thick collections of fibrous strands form the radiating structure.

Comment

In spite of the large size of this tumor, there is no skin thickening or retraction.

Conclusion

Mammographically benign lesion. Typical picture of sclerosing duct hyperplasia (radial scar).

Histology

Sclerosing duct hyperplasia. No evidence of malignancy.
Fig. 62 C: Operative specimen photograph.

Fig. 62 C see Color Plate I after p. 136.

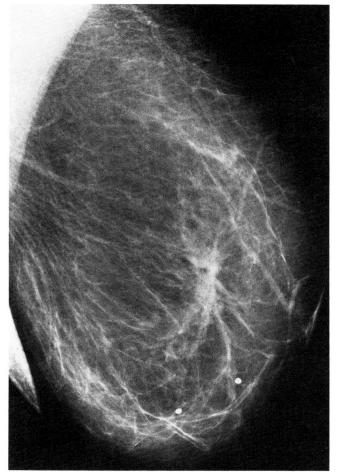

A

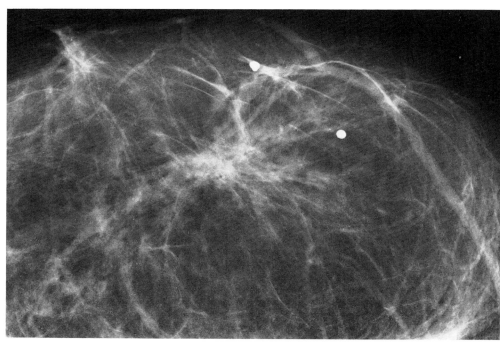

B

63

Asymptomatic 69-year-old woman. First screening study.

Physical Examination

No palpable tumor.

Mammography

Fig. 63 A: Left breast, detailed view of the medio-lateral oblique projection. There is a large stellate tumor in the upper half of the breast.
Fig. 63 B & C: Left breast, magnification views, medio-lateral oblique and cranio-caudal projections.

Analysis (best on the magnification views)

Stellate lesion. No solid tumor center. Numerous longitudinal, oval and circular radiolucencies within the tumor. The radiating structure consists of thick collections of connective tissue strands bunched together. Alternating with them are radiolucent linear structures parallel to these strands. No associated calcifications.

Conclusion

Typical mammographic appearance of sclerosing duct hyperplasia (radial scar).

Comment

Even with such a large, superficial lesion, no tumor could be palpated. This supports the diagnosis of sclerosing duct hyperplasia.

Histology

Sclerosing duct hyperplasia. No evidence of malignancy.

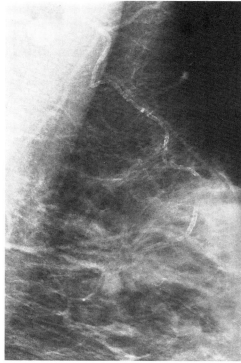

A

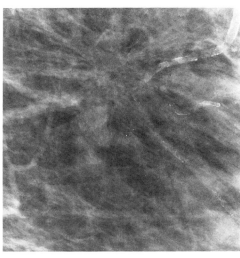

B

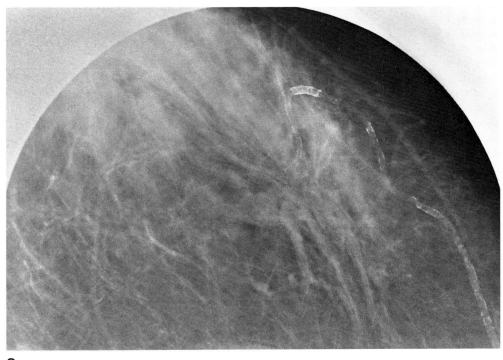

C

64

Age 52, referred for pain in the right breast.

Physical Examination

No palpable tumor in either breast.

Mammography

Fig. 64 A: Right breast, medio-lateral oblique projection. 7 cm from the nipple at coordinate A1 there is a stellate lesion.

Fig. 64 B: Right breast, cranio-caudal projection. The stellate lesion is seen at coordinate A1.

Fig. 64 C: Right breast, enlarged view of the medio-lateral projection.

Analysis

Stellate lesion. No solid tumor center. The appearance of the lesion changes remarkably with the projection. The radiating structure consists of connective tissue strands bunched together. Between the bunches there are linear translucencies.

Conclusion

Typical mammographic appearance of sclerosing duct hyperplasia (radial scar).

Histology

Sclerosing duct hyperplasia. No evidence of malignancy.

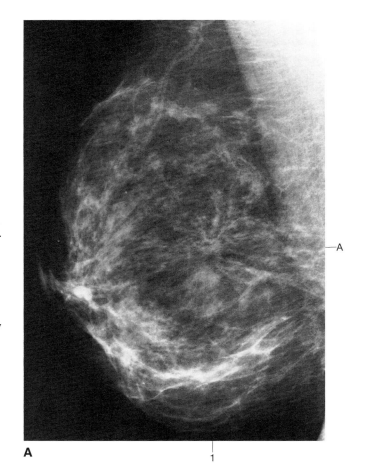

A

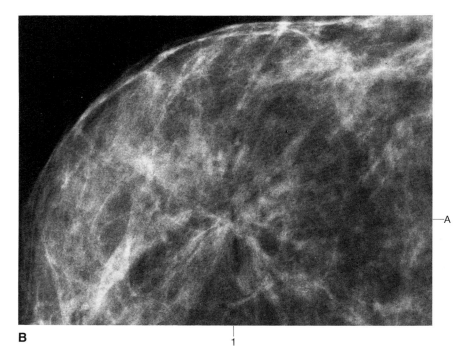

B

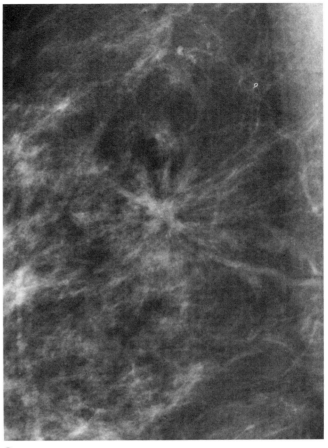

c

65

Asymptomatic 63-year-old woman. First screening examination.

Physical Examination

No palpable tumor in the breasts.

Mammography

Fig. 65 A: Right breast, medio-lateral oblique projection.
Fig. 65 B: Right breast, cranio-caudal projection.
Fig. 65 C: Coned-down view of the cranio-caudal projection.
A stellate tumor is seen 6 cm from the nipple in the lateral half of the breast. No associated calcifications.

Conclusion

Typical mammographic picture of a small infiltrating carcinoma. Solid tumor mass, radiating spicules.

Histology

Tubular carcinoma. Size 6 mm. No axillary metastases.

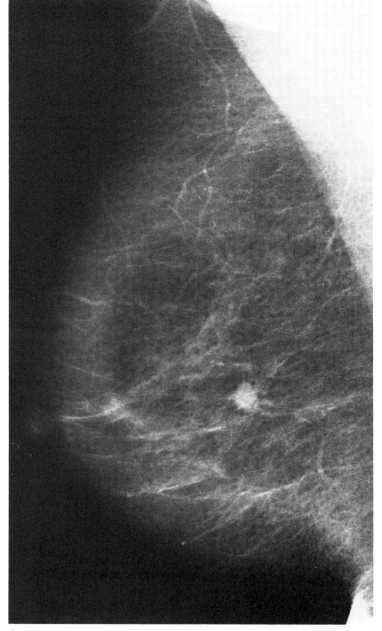

A

B

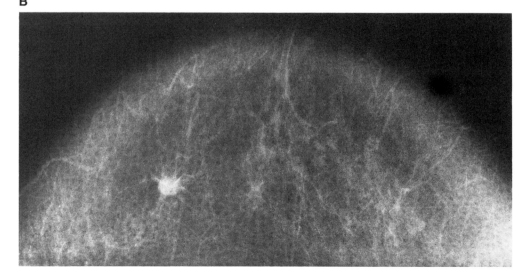

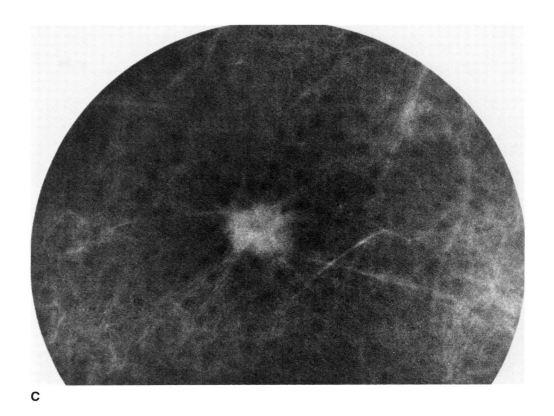

c

66

Asymptomatic woman, age 66. First screening study.

Physical Examination

No palpable tumor.

Mammography

Fig. 66 A: Right breast, medio-lateral oblique projection: There is a tumor with a radiating structure 9 cm from the nipple. Calcifications are scattered throughout the breast.

Analysis of the Tumor

Form: stellate, no central tumor mass; instead, the center is radiolucent; the spicules are fine, long and bunched together in thick collections like sheaves of wheat
Size: large, difficult to determine, approximately 5 × 4 cm

Conclusion

The combination of the above mentioned mammographic signs is characteristic of sclerosing duct hyperplasia (radial scar).

Analysis of the Calcifications

Form: elongated, smooth-bordered, some needle-like
Density: high, uniform
Size: within dilated ducts
Distribution: along the course of the ducts

Conclusion

Typical picture of calcifications resulting from plasma cell mastitis.

Comment

Benign tumor and benign-type calcifications unrelated to each other. Although the mammographic picture is characteristic of sclerosing duct hyperplasia, detailed histologic examination is necessary as in all stellate lesions. The tumor was excised *in toto*. Fig. 66 B: Specimen photograph. Note the thick radiating connective tissue strands. There appears to be a hole in the center of the lesion corresponding

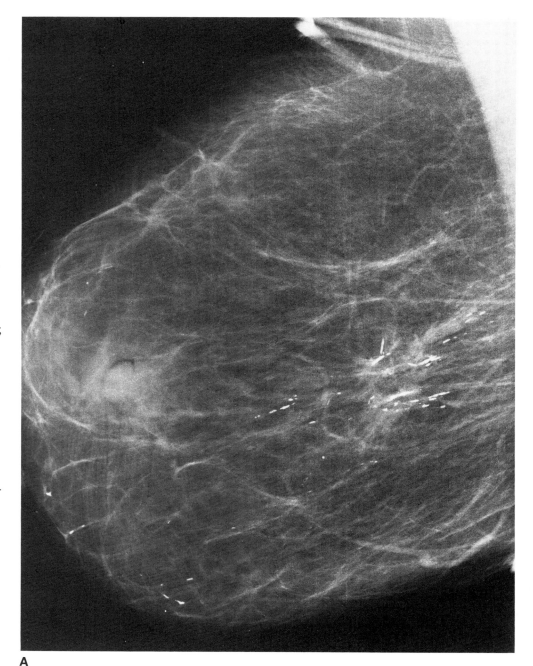

A

Fig. 66 B see Color Plate I, after p. 136.

to the radiolucent center on the mammogram.

Histology

Sclerosing duct hyperplasia. No evidence of malignancy.
Fig. 66 C: Right breast (same case 6 months later). A palpable tumor has developed at the site of operation. Medio-lateral-oblique projection: the palpable tumor corresponds to the large, stellate density on the mammogram. Re-operation.

Histology

Traumatic fat necrosis. No evidence of malignancy.

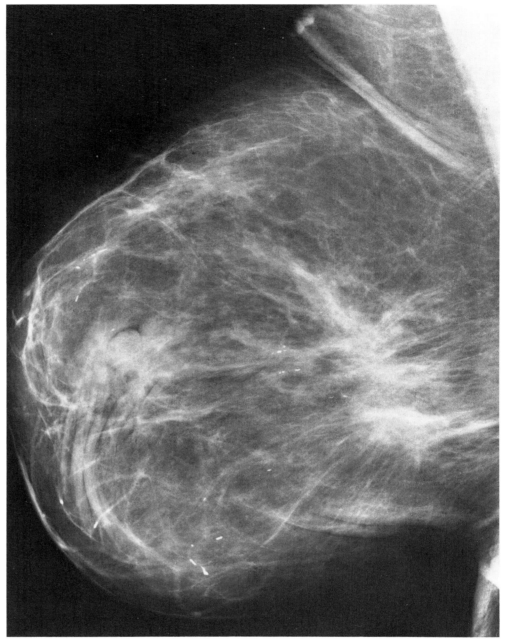

C

67

Age 63.

Physical Examination

A hard, freely movable lump was palpated in the upper inner quadrant of the right breast. Not suspicious for malignancy.

Mammography

Fig. 67 A & B: Right breast, mediolateral oblique and cranio-caudal projections. There is a large stellate tumor in the upper inner quadrant of the breast with associated calcifications. Fig. 67 C: Coned-down compression view, cranio-caudal projection.

Analysis

The radiating structure consists of thick collections of connective tissue strands. There are coarse calcifications at the center of the stellate lesion.

Conclusion

This radiating structure differs from that seen with malignant tumors. The associated calcifications are of the benign type. This large lesion, although superficial, does not cause skin changes. It is mammographically benign, consistent with sclerosing duct hyperplasia (radial scar).

Histology

Sclerosing duct hyperplasia. No evidence of malignancy.

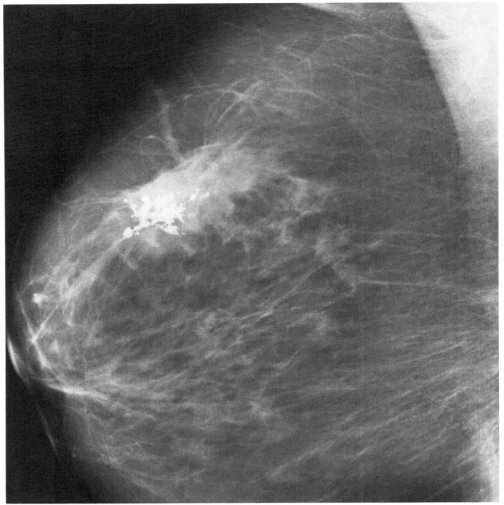

A

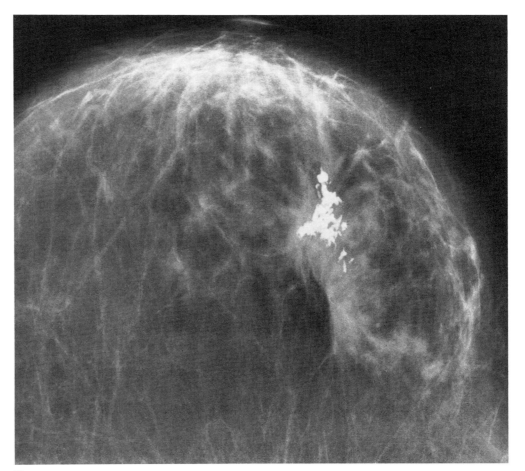

B

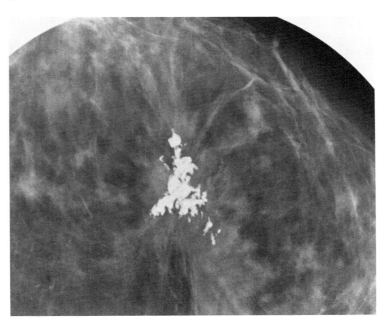

C

68

Age 45, operated for a large cyst in the right breast.

Mammography

Fig. 68 A: Right breast, cranio-caudal projection preoperatively. There is a large cyst in the medial half of the breast.

Fig. 68 B: Right breast, cranio-caudal projection 6 months after operation. A large, stellate lesion is seen at the site of operation. No associated calcifications.

Fig. 68 C: Right breast, cranio-caudal projection two years after operation. Reduction in size oft the stellate lesion.

Analysis

Center of the lesion (Fig. 68 C): This has become so indistinct that it is difficult to locate. There are circular and oval translucencies in the lesion (arrows).

Radiating structure: Much less apparent.

Conclusion

Traumatic fat necrosis. This case demonstrates the typical appearance and regression of this lesion.

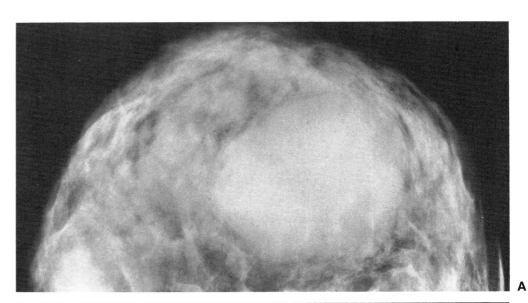

A

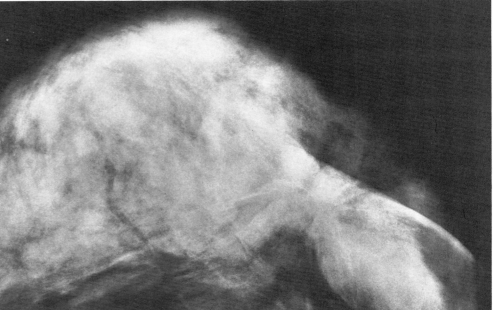

B

C

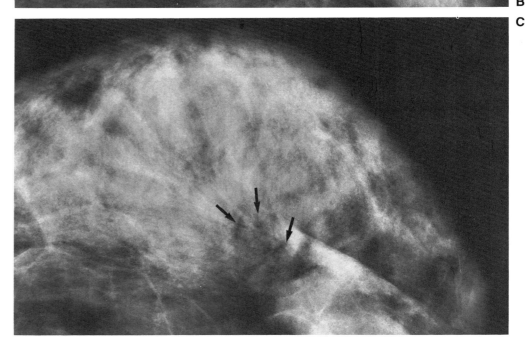

69

Age 67. First screening study. History of right breast operation 25 years earlier with retraction of skin and a thick scar at the operative site, unchanged in recent years.

Mammography

Fig. 69 A & B: Right breast, mediolateral oblique and detailed view of the cranio-caudal projection. There is a stellate tumor in the lower outer quadrant with central calcifications and associated skin retraction.

Analysis

Tumor center: Definite central mass, but it contains lucent areas. The appearance of the tumor changes with projection.
Radiating structure: On the craniocaudal projection (Fig. 69 B), radiolucent linear structures form part of the stellate lesion. The overlying skin is thickened and retracted.
Calcifications: Coarse, highly dense, centrally located, mammographically of the benign type.

Comment

A stellate lesion on the mammogram which changes its appearance with projection and contains central translucencies (either linear, oval or circular) is characteristic of the cancer-mimicking benign stellate lesions: sclerosing duct hyperplasia, and the stellate form of traumatic fat necrosis. The history may help in differentiation, as in this case.

Histology

Foreign body granuloma.

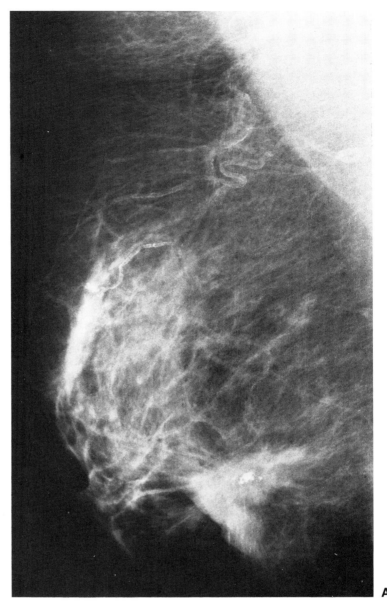

A

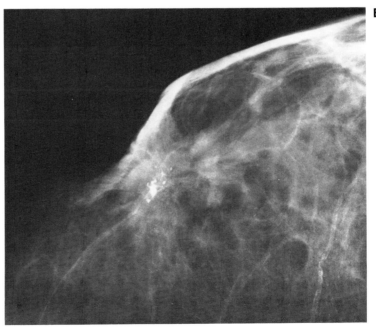

B

70

Asymptomatic 70-year-old woman. First screening examination.

Physical Examination

No palpable tumor in the breasts.

Mammography

Fig. 70 A & B & C: Voluminous right breast which required 3 films for one medio-lateral oblique projection.
Fig. 70 D: Right breast, cranio-caudal projection. A small tumor is seen at coordinate A1 in these four mammograms.
Fig. 70 E: Microfocus magnification view, cranio-caudal projection. The tumor is seen at coordinate A1.

Analysis

Central tumor mass with long radiating spicules. No associated calcifications. Mammographically malignant tumor.
Fig. 70 F: Specimen photograph.

Histology

Infiltrating ductal carcinoma, size 7 mm. No axillary lymph node metastases.

Fig. 70 F see Color Plate I, after p. 136.

Comment

There are a number of other radiopaque, poorly-defined parenchymal structures in this breast. Only the tumor, with its radiating spicular structure, is abnormal.

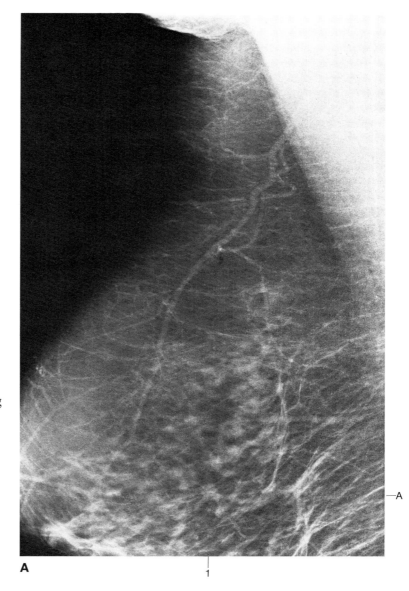

A   1

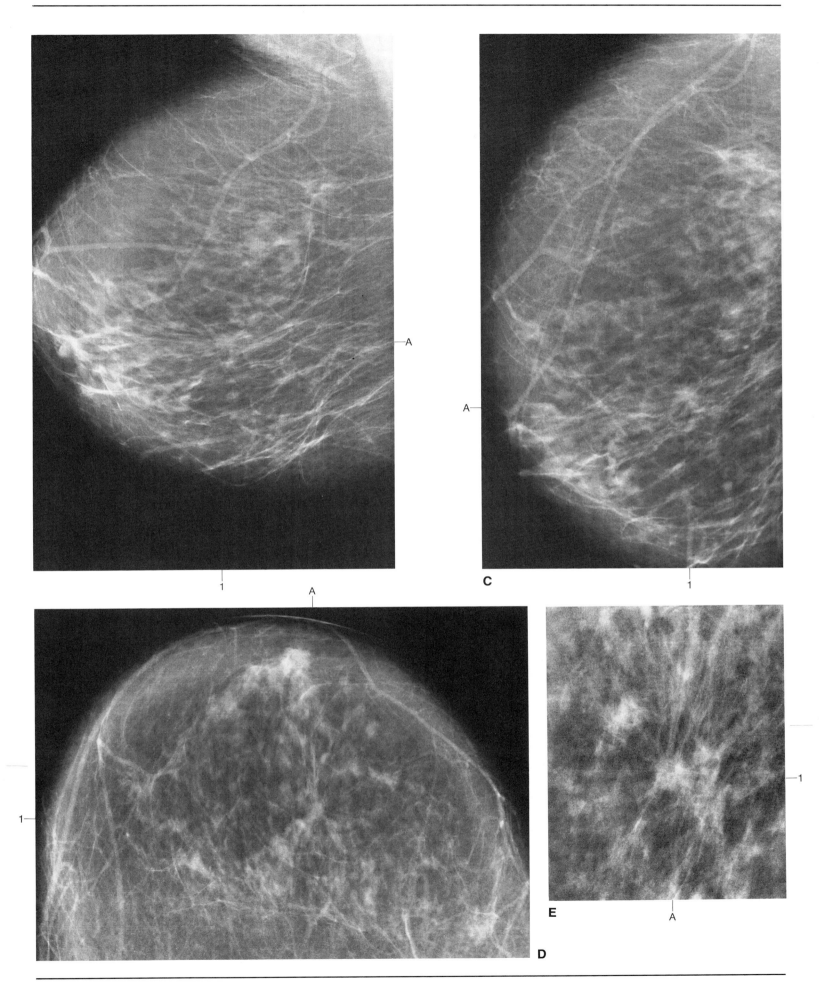

71

Age 60.

Physical Examination

3 cm lump detected laterally in the left breast, clinically suspicious for malignancy.

Mammography

Fig. 71 A & B: Right and left breasts, medio-lateral oblique projections.
Fig. 71 C: Left breast, cranio-caudal projection.

Fig. 71 D & E: Coned-down compression views, cranio-caudal projection. At coordinate A1 in Fig. 71 B & C there is a 2 cm stellate tumor. No associated calcifications.

Analysis

(Best on the coned-down compression views)

Stellate tumor with a central tumor mass, size 15 × 15 mm. The spicules are short. The overlying parenchyma is dense and obscures much of the tumor.

Conclusion

Mammographically malignant tumor.

Comment

This case is a problem in perception rather than in analysis. The tumor can be detected on the medio-lateral oblique projection by oblique masking, caudal aspect (see Chapter II). Retraction of the posterior parenchymal border on the cranio-caudal projection (Fig. 71 C) produces the "tent-sign" (see Chapter II).

Histology

Infiltrating ductal carcinoma. No axillary lymph node metastases.

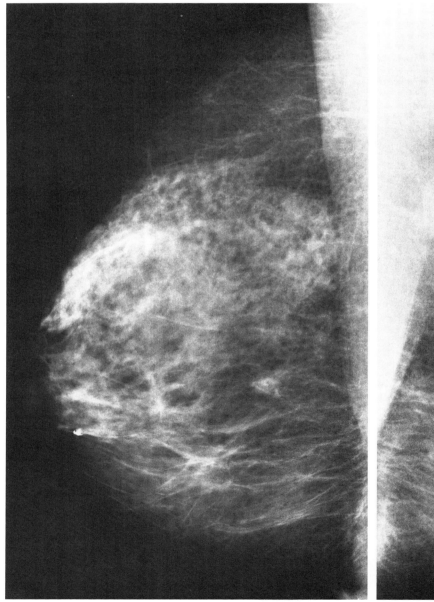

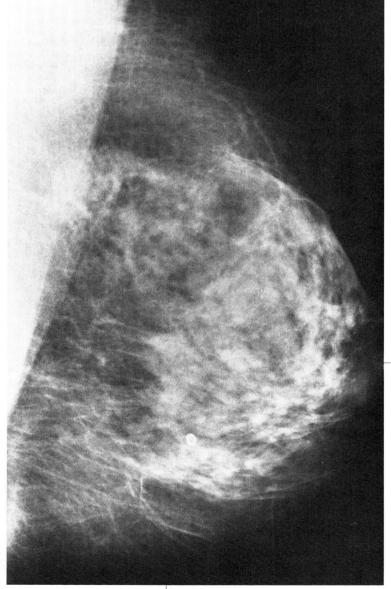

A

B

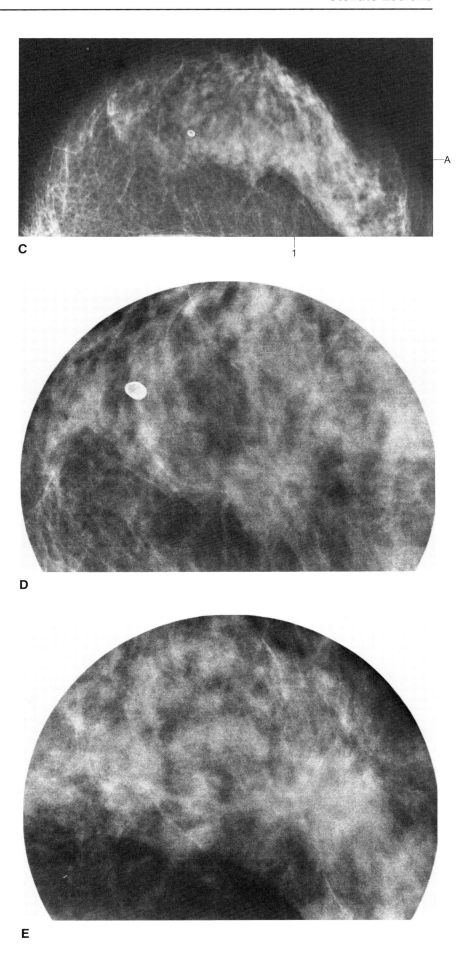

C

D

E

72

Asymptomatic 71-year-old-woman. First screening examination.

Physical Examination

No palpable tumor.

Mammography

Fig. 72 A & B: Right and left breasts, medio-lateral oblique projections. Normal right breast. At coordinate A1 there is a small stellate tumor with no associated calcifications.
Fig. 72 C: Left breast, cranio-caudal projection.
Fig. 72 D & E: Enlarged coned-down compression views, cranio-caudal and latero-medial projections.
Fig. 72 F: Operative specimen.

Analysis

Form: stellate; small tumor mass with surrounding spicules
Size: less than 10 mm

Conclusion

Mammographically malignant tumor.

Histology

Infiltrating ductal carcinoma. No axillary lymph node metastases.

Comment

This case represents a problem in perception, which can be solved by horizontal masking, cranial aspect (see Chapter II).

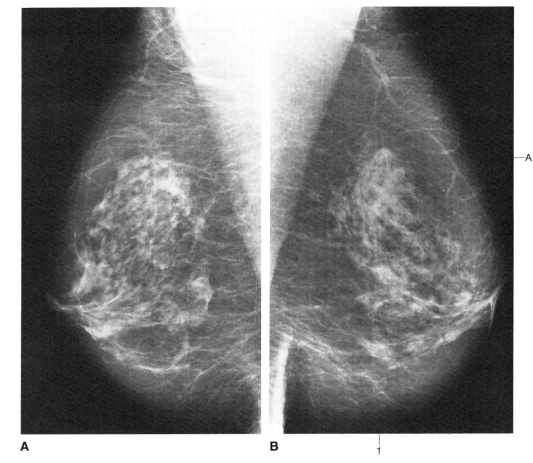

A   B

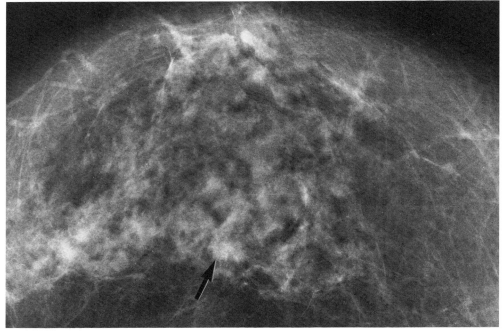

C

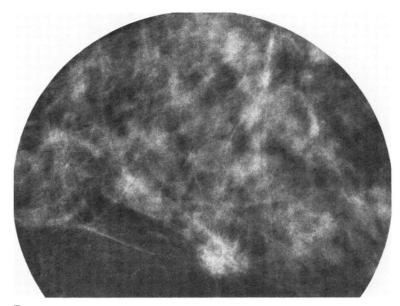

D

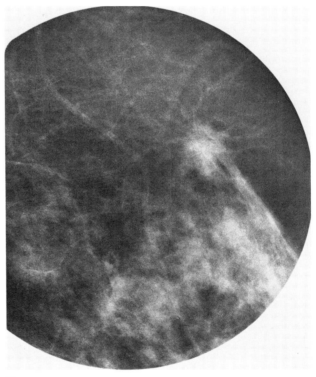

E

Fig. 72 F see Color Plate I, after
p. 136.

73

Asymptomatic 68-year-old woman.
First screening study.

Physical Examination

With knowledge of the mammogram a
tumor could be vaguely palpated in the
upper outer quadrant of the right
breast.

Mammography

Fig. 73 A: Right breast, medio-lateral
oblique projection. A tumor is seen at
coordinate A1. There are coarse calcifications not associated with the
tumor 4 cm from the nipple.
Fig. 73 B: Left breast, medio-lateral
oblique projection. No mammographic
abnormality.

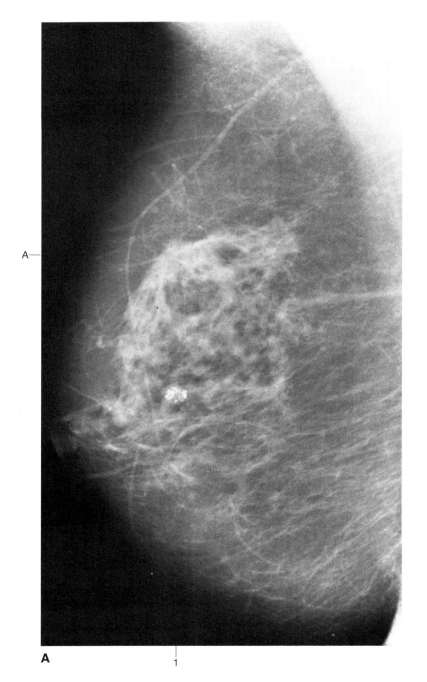

A
1

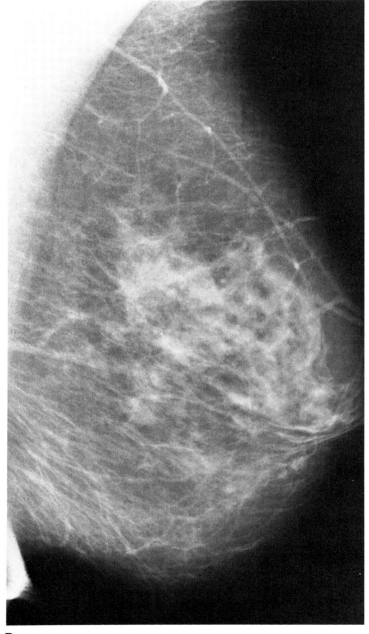

B

Fig. 73 C: Right breast, detailed view of the cranio-caudal projection. The tumor is located at coordinate A1.
Fig. 73 D: Right breast, microfocus magnification view, medio-lateral oblique projection. There is a stellate tumor with a distinct central mass, size approximately 10 mm, surrounded by long, sharp spicules.

Conclusion

Typical mammographic appearance of a stellate malignant tumor. The calcifications 4 cm from the nipple are coarse and of the benign type, typical of a hyalinized fibroadenoma.

Histology

Infiltrating ductal carcinoma, size 10 mm. No axillary lymph node metastases.

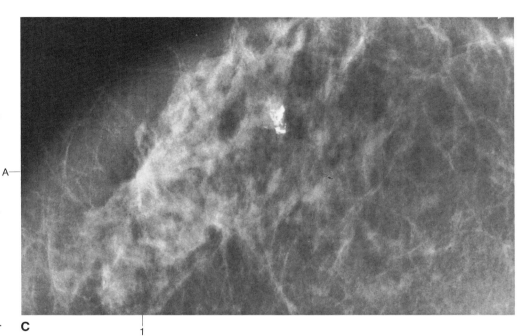

C

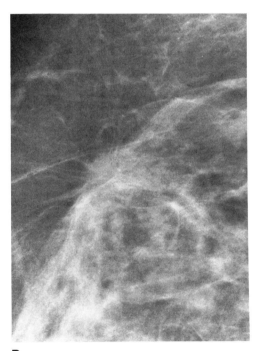

D

74

Asymptomatic 57-year-old woman. First screening study.

Physical Examination

No palpable tumor in the breasts.

Mammography

Fig. 74 A & B: Right and left breast, medio-lateral oblique projections. A small tumor is seen at coordinate A1 in the upper outer quadrant of the left breast.
Fig. 74 C: Left breast, cranio-caudal projection.
Fig. 74 D: Magnification view in the cranio-caudal projection.
Small stellate tumor with a central tumor mass, mammographically malignant.

Histology

Infiltrating ductal carcinoma, size less than 10 mm. No axillary metastases.

Comment

This tumor is difficult to locate on the medio-lateral oblique projection. Oblique masking, cranial aspect, helps reveal the tumor (Fig. VIII B, Chapter II). The density seen at coord. A2 corresponds to the so-called desmoplastic reaction (connective tissue proliferation in the vicinity of the malignant tumor).

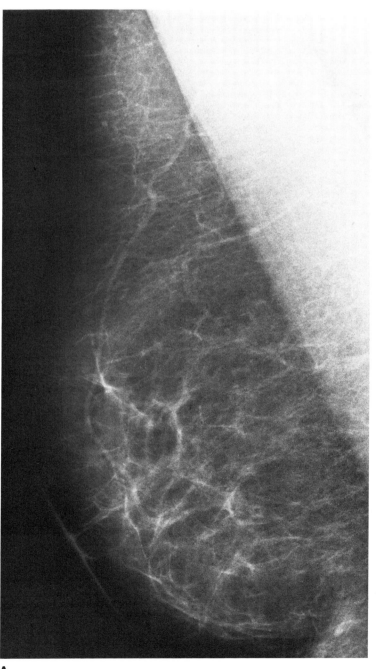

A

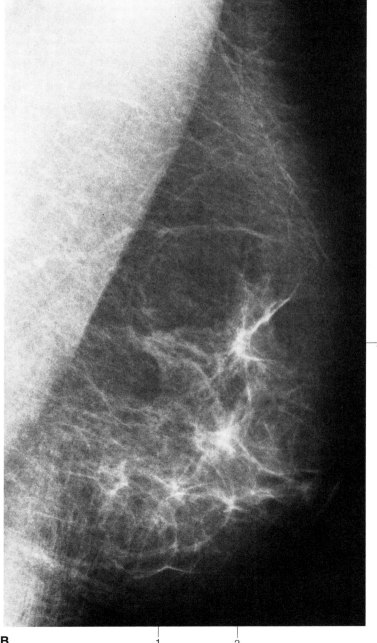

B

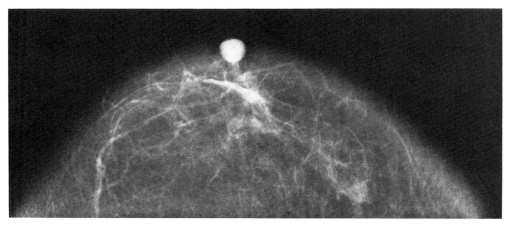

C

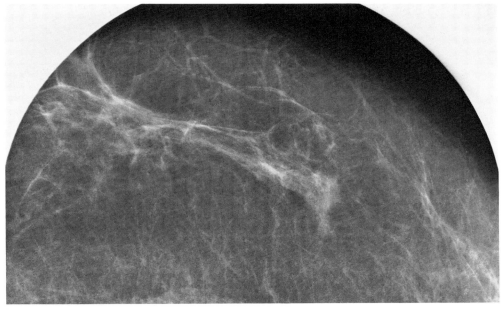

D

75

65-year-old, asymptomatic woman. First screening study.

Physical Examination

No palpable tumor in the breasts.

Mammography

Fig. 75 A & B: Left breast, medio-lateral oblique and cranio-caudal projections.
A small tumor is seen in the upper outer quadrant, 9 cm from the nipple, at coordinate A1.
Fig. 75 C & D: Microfocus magnification views, medio-lateral oblique and cranio-caudal projections.

Analysis

Stellate tumor, less than 10 mm in size with a radiating structure.
Mammographic diagnosis: malignant tumor.
Fig. 75 E: Operative specimen photograph, see Color Plate I, after p. 136.

Histology

Infiltrative ductal carcinoma. Size 9 mm. No axillary lymph node metastases.

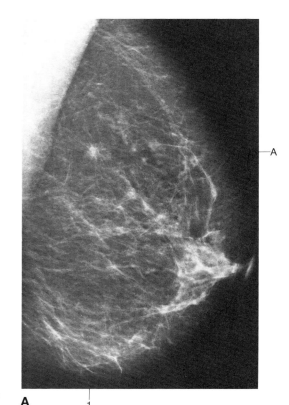

A

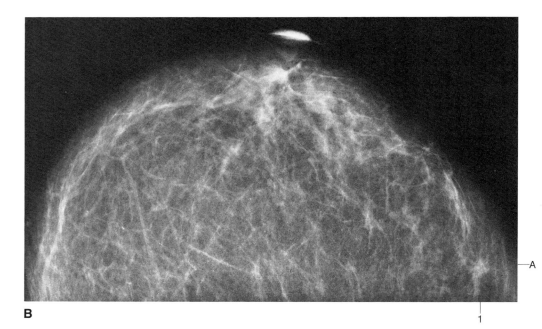

B

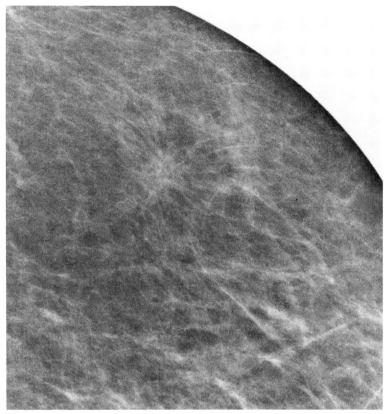

C

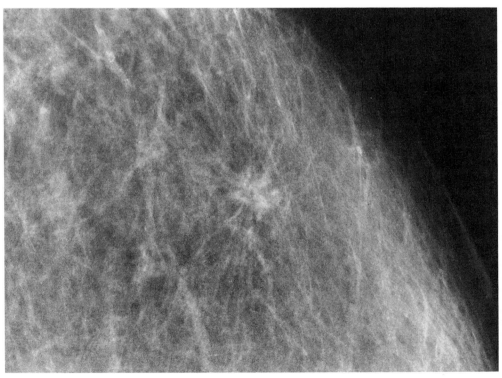

D

76

73-year-old woman, asymptomatic.
First screening study.

Physical Examination

No palpable tumor in the breasts.

Mammography

Fig. 76 A & B: Right and left breasts, medio-lateral oblique projections. There is a stellate tumor at coordinate A1 in the right breast.
Fig. 76 C: Right breast, cranio-caudal projection. The tumor is seen at coordinate A1.

Fig. 76 D: Coned-down compression view in the cranio-caudal projection.
Fig. 76 E: Right breast. Enlarged view in the medio-lateral projection. The tumor is located at coordinate A1.

Analysis

Form: stellate; small tumor mass with surrounding spicules; no associated calcifications
Size: less than 10 mm

Conclusion

Mammographically malignant tumor.

Comment

The smaller the stellate tumor, the greater the difficulty in perception. The tumor can be detected on the

medio-lateral oblique projection using oblique masking, cranial aspect (see Chapter II).
Fig. 76 F: Operative specimen photograph, see Color Plate II, after p. 136.

Histology

Infiltrating ductal carcinoma, maximum diameter 10 mm. No axillary metastases.

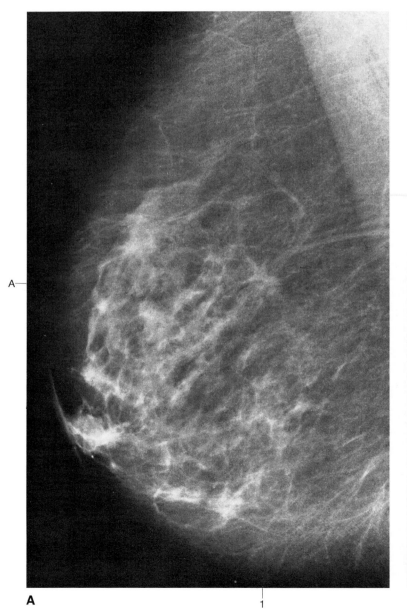

A

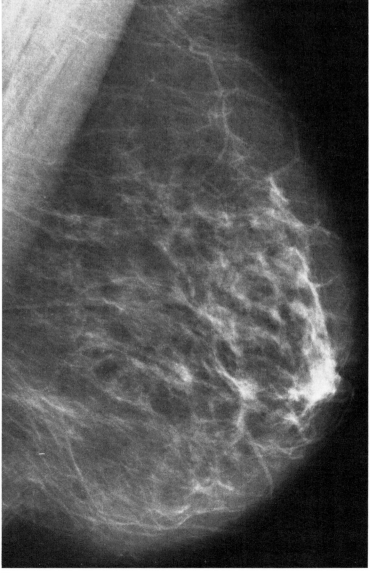

B

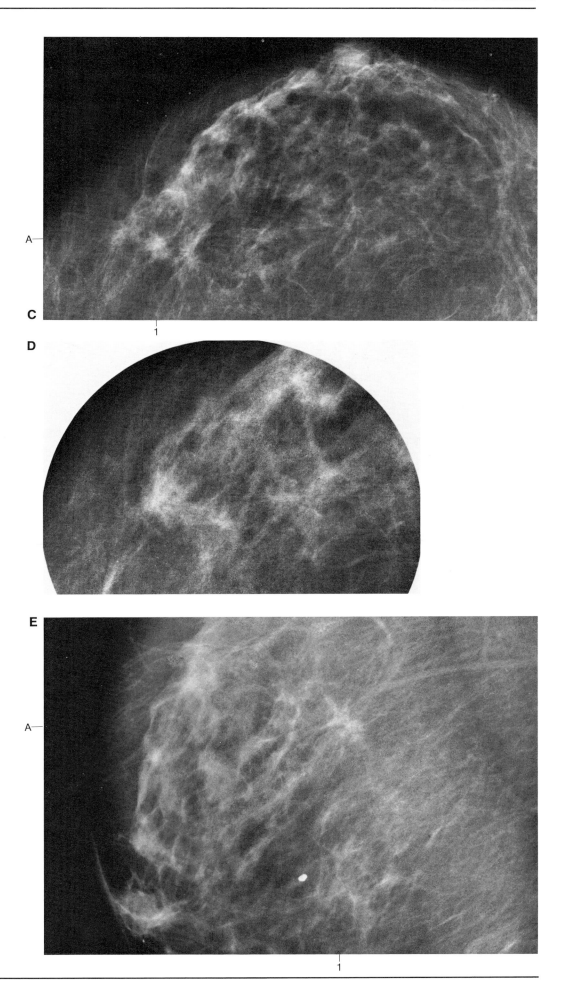

77

61-year-old woman, asymptomatic.
First screening study.

Physical Examination

No palpable tumor in the breasts.

Mammography

Fig. 77 A: Left breast, medio-lateral oblique projection. At coordinate A1 there is parenchymal distortion.
Fig. 77 B: Left breast, cranio-caudal projection. There is a centrally located stellate tumor 6 cm from the nipple.
Fig. 77 C: Left breast, microfocus magnification view in the cranio-caudal projection.
Fig. 77 D: Operative specimen radiograph.

Analysis

Stellate lesion. No definite central tumor mass. Long, fine spicules form the radiating structure. No associated calcifications.

Conclusion

Typical mammographic appearance of sclerosing duct hyperplasia.

Histology

Infiltrating ductal carcinoma. No axillary metastases.

Comment

As mentioned in Chapters V and VIII, the final diagnosis of stellate lesions can be made only by histology.

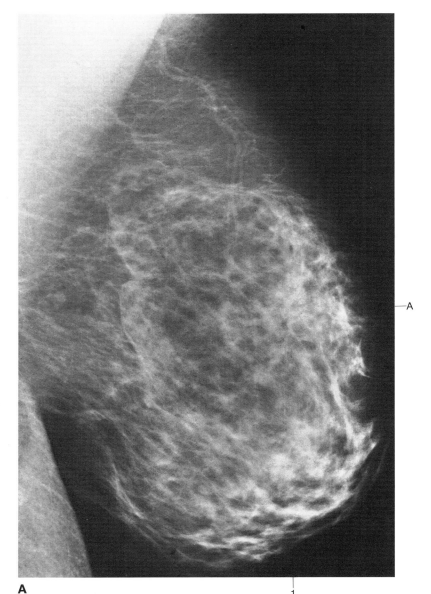

A

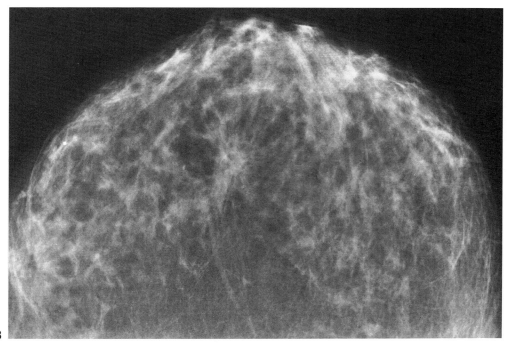

B

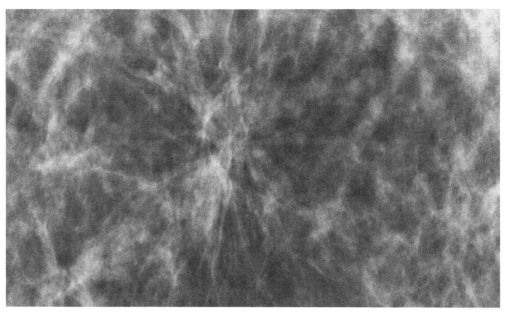

C

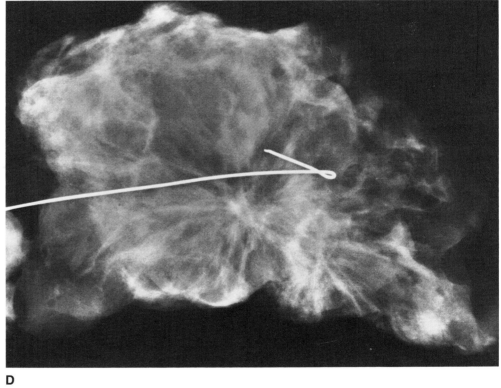

D

78

64-year-old woman, asymptomatic. First screening study.

Physical Examination

No palpable tumor in the breasts.

Mammography

Fig. 78 A & B: Right and left breasts, medio-lateral oblique projections. At coordinate A1 in the left breast there is a small stellate tumor. Right breast normal.

Fig. 78 C: Left breast, cranio-caudal projection. The tumor is seen at coordinate A1.

Fig. 78 D: Left breast, coned-down compression view in the cranio-caudal projection. The tumor is seen superimposed on the calcified artery.

Analysis

Form: stellate; central tumor mass with surrounding short spicules, best seen in the coned-down compression view

Size: less than 10 mm

Conclusion

Mammographically malignant tumor.

Histology

Infiltrating ductal carcinoma, maximum diameter 7 mm. No axillary lymph node metastases.

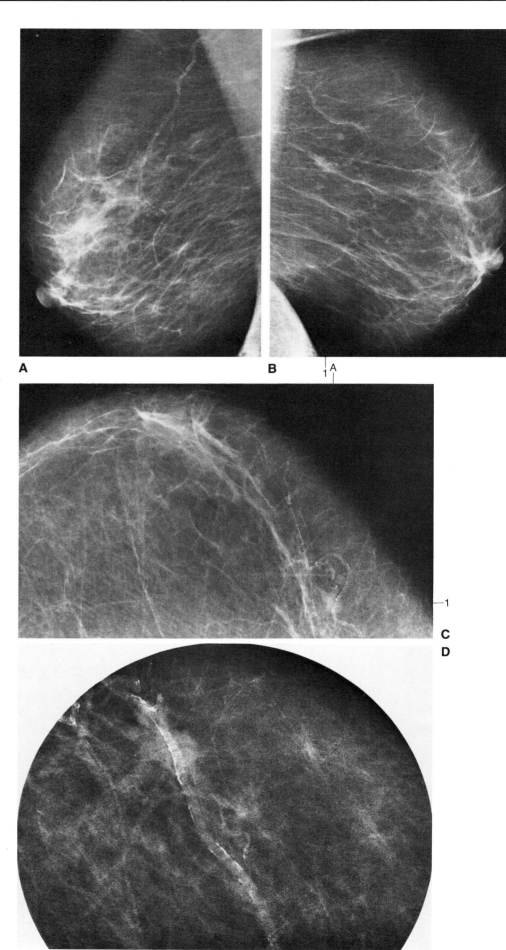

79

70-year-old woman, asymptomatic.
First screening examination.

Physical Examination

No palpable tumor in the breasts.

Mammography

Fig. 79 A: Right breast, medio-lateral oblique projection. A small stellate tumor is seen at coordinate A1.
Fig. 79 B: Right breast, cranio-caudal projection. The stellate lesion is seen at coordinate A1.
Fig. 79 C: Coned-down compression view of the tumor in the medio-lateral oblique projection.

Analysis

Form: stellate lesion with a central tumor mass
Radiating structure: short spicules
Size: less than 1 cm

Conclusion

Mammographically highly suspicious for malignancy.

Histology

Infiltrating ductal carcinoma, size 6 × 6 mm. No axillary lymph node metastases.

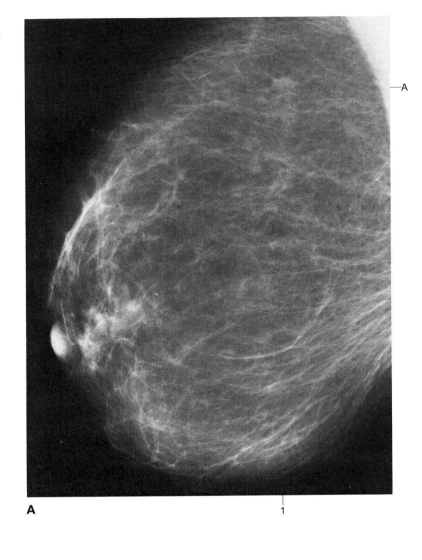

A   1

B   **C**

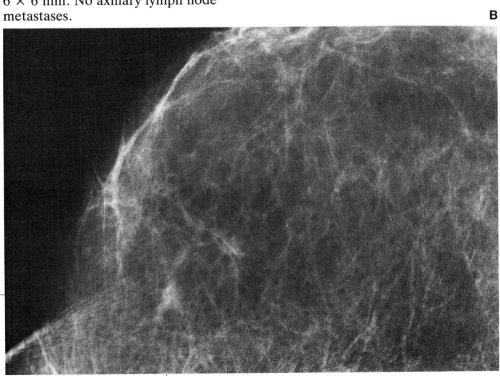

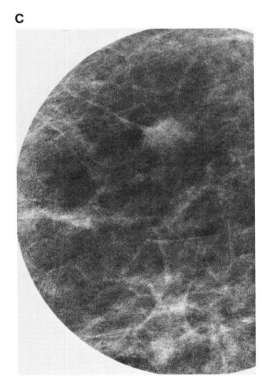

80

Age 44, referred for mammography for a palpable tumor in the upper outer quadrant of the left breast.

Physical Examination

2 × 2 cm hard lump in the upper outer quadrant of the left breast. No skin changes. Suspicious for malignancy.

Mammography

Fig. 80 A: Left breast, medio-lateral oblique projection. There is parenchymal retraction at coordinate A1. No associated calcifications (see Fig. XII).
Fig. 80 B: Left breast, cranio-caudal projection. There is parenchymal distortion at coordinate A1. Tent sign (Fig. XI).
Fig. 80 C: Left breast, coned-down compression view, cranio-caudal projection.

Analysis (best on the coned-down compression view)

Stellate tumor with a central tumor mass surrounded by numerous spicules. Mammographically malignant tumor.

Histology

Infiltrating comedo carcinoma with axillary lymph node metastases.

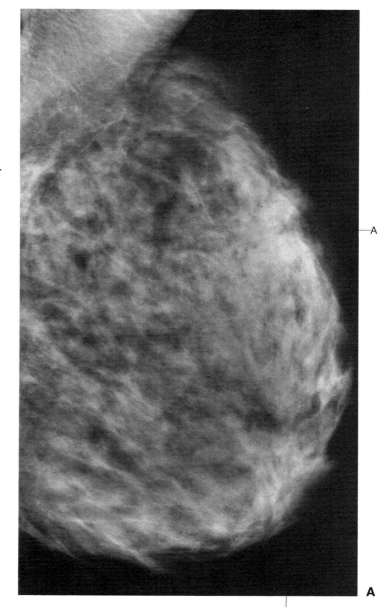

A

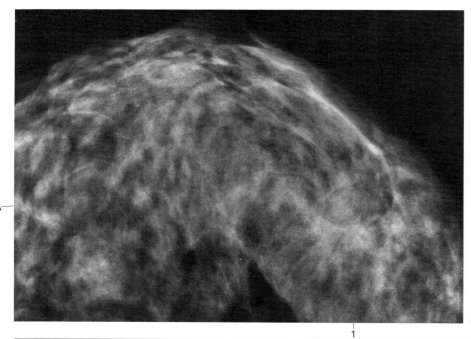

B

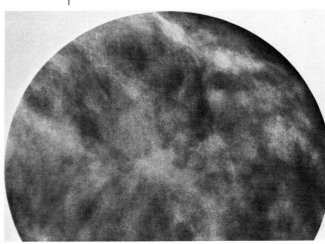

C

81

46-year-old asymptomatic woman. First screening study.

Physical Examination

No palpable tumor in the breasts.

Mammography

Fig. 81 A: Left breast, medio-lateral oblique projection. A stellate tumor is seen 8 cm from the nipple in the upper half of the breast.
Fig. 81 B: Left breast, enlarged view of the medio-lateral oblique projection.

Analysis

Stellate tumor. An oval translucency is seen near the center of the lesion. The stellate structure is formed by radiating radiolucent linear structures. The calcifications are very faint.

Conclusion

Typical mammographic appearance of sclerosing duct hyperplasia (radial scar).

Histology

Sclerosing duct hyperplasia. No evidence of malignancy.

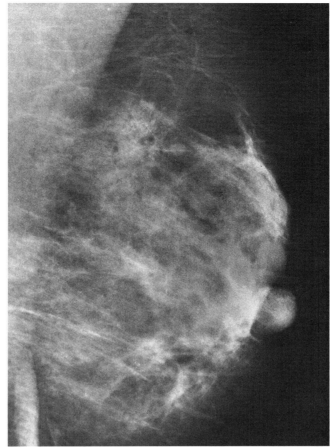

A

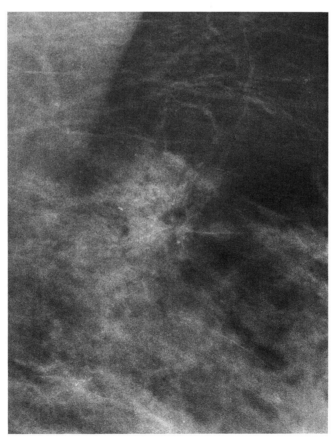

B

82

42-year-old woman, asymptomatic. First screening examination.

Physical Examination

No palpable tumor in the breasts.

Mammography

Fig. 82 A & B: Right and left breasts, medio-lateral oblique projections. At coordinate A1, in the right breast, there is a small stellate tumor.
Fig. 82 C: Right breast, cranio-caudal projection, with the tumor at coordinate A1.

Fig. 82 D: Right breast, microfocus magnification view, cranio-caudal projection.

Analysis

Stellate lesion. The appearance varies with the projection. No central tumor mass. Long, fine spicules. No associated calcifications.

Conclusion

Although the central lucencies are not present in this case, the absence of a solid tumor center and the relatively long, fine spicules are the most important diagnostic factors supporting the mammographic diagnosis of sclerosing duct hyperplasia (radial scar). Differentiation cannot be reliably made from a small stellate malignant tumor.

Histology

Sclerosing duct hyperplasia. No evidence of malignancy.

Comment

This tumor is difficult to perceive. Oblique masking, cranial aspect, helps to locate it (Fig. 82 E & F).

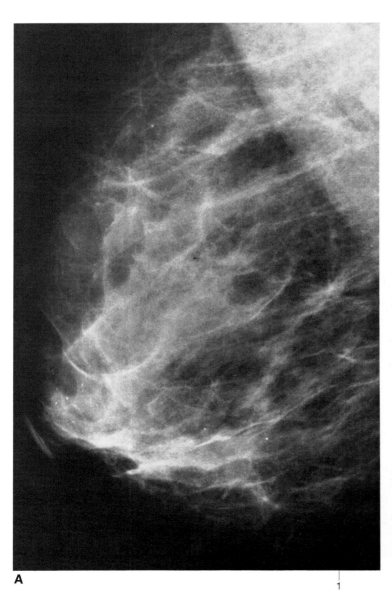

A

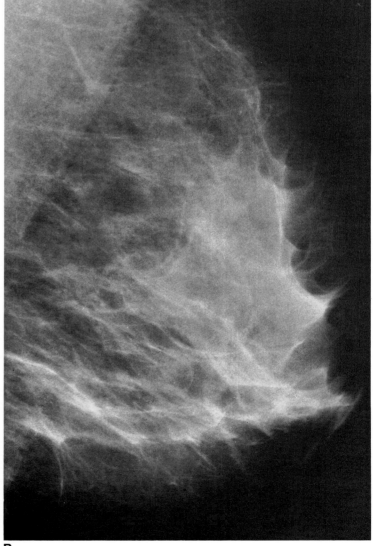

B

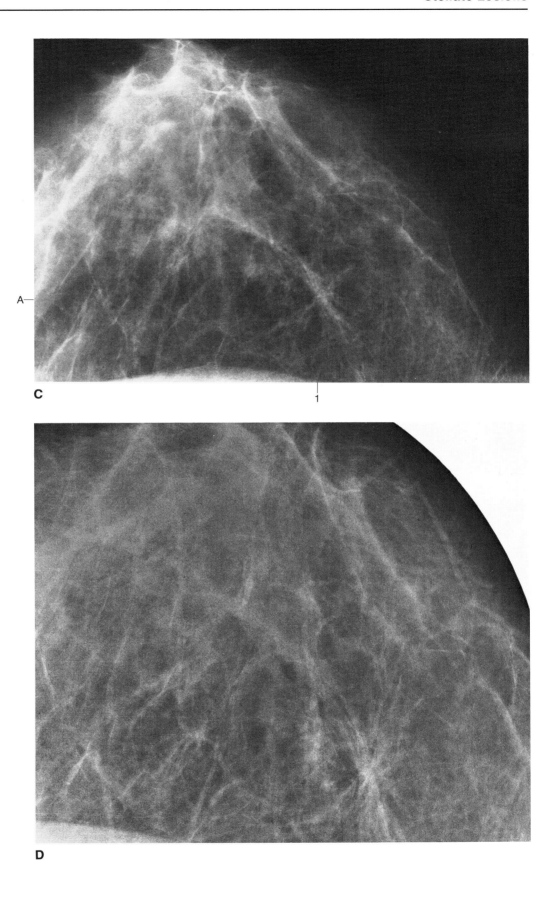

C

A—

1

D

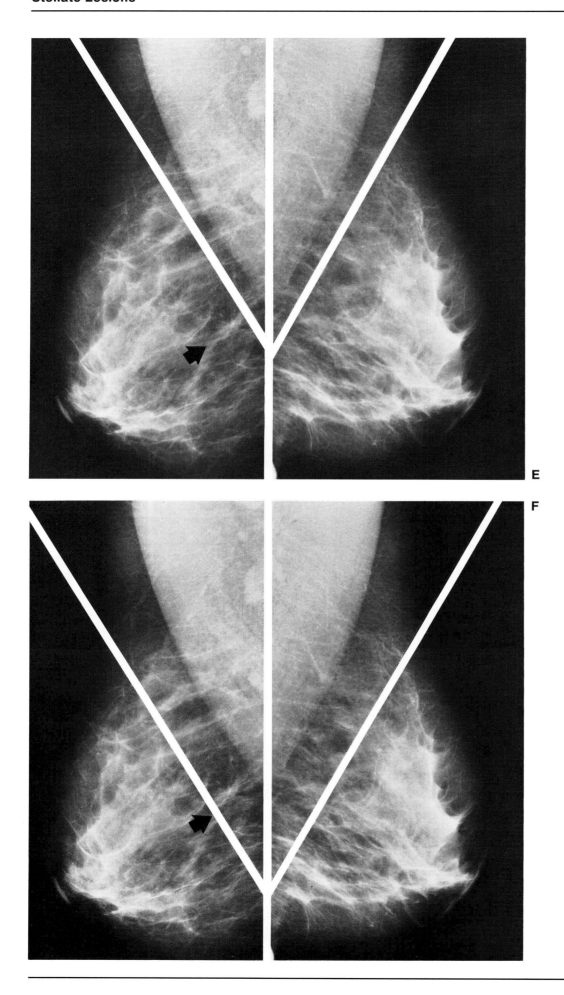

E

F

83

41-year-old woman, asymptomatic.
First screening examination.

Physical Examination

No palpable tumor in the breasts.

Mammography

Fig. 83 A: Left breast, cranio-caudal
projection. There is a tumor with
radiating structure in the central portion of the breast. No associated calcifications.
Fig. 83 B & C: Microfocus magnification views, cranio-caudal and medio-
lateral oblique projections.

Analysis

A large, radiating structure, consisting
of numerous long and fine spicules
interspersed with linear radiolucencies
(arrows). There is a remarkable difference in the appearance of Fig. 83 B
and C.

Conclusion

Mammographic picture sclerosing duct
hyperplasia (radial scar).

Histology

Sclerosing duct hyperplasia.
Thorough histologic examination
revealed an associated intraductal
cancer with minimal infiltration.

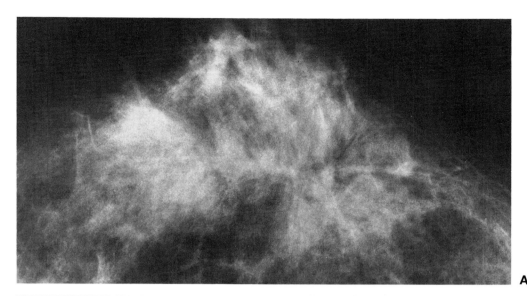

A

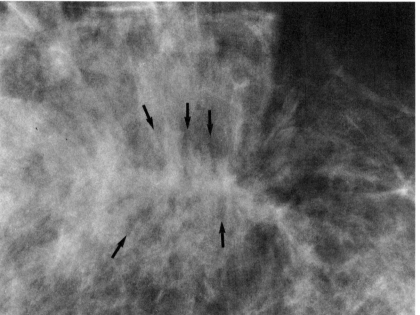

B

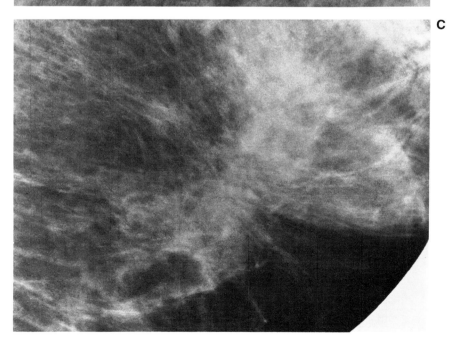

C

84

Age 41, right breast operated four months earlier for a benign lesion. Screening examination.

Mammography

Fig. 84 A & B: Right breast, medio-lateral oblique and cranio-caudal projections. There is a stellate lesion in the upper inner quadrant with no associated calcifications.

Analysis

Tumor Center: There are several radiolucent areas within the indistinct tumor center.
Radiating structure: Very fine, long, low density spicules. The skin is slightly retracted at the site of operation.

Conclusion

The history of recent breast surgery confirms the diagnosis of traumatic fat necrosis with considerable certainty. The mammographic description is typical of the stellate form of traumatic fat necrosis.

Repeat Mammography

Fig. 84 C: Right breast, medio-lateral oblique projection, 2 years later. There is nearly complete resolution of the stellate lesion with a small crater at the operative site.

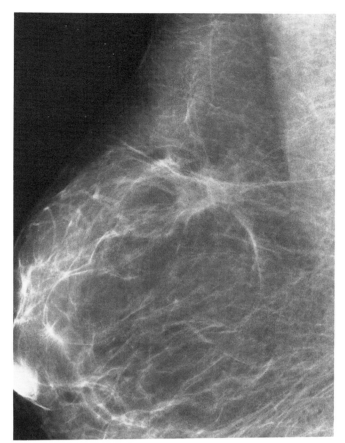

A

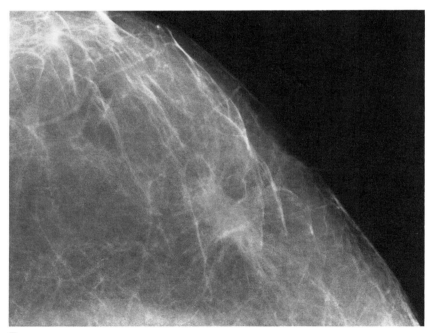

B

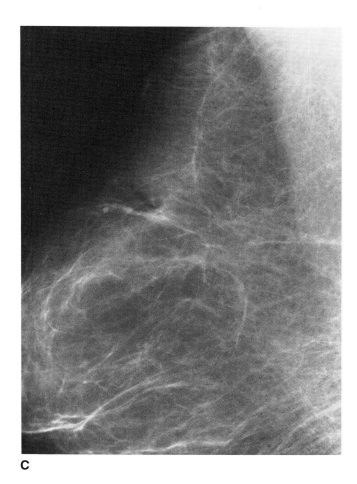

c

85

61-year-old asymptomatic woman. First screening study.

Physical Examination

No palpable tumor in the breasts.

Mammography

Fig. 85 A & B: Left breast, mediolateral oblique and cranio-caudal projections. At coordinate A1 a solitary, non-calcified tumor is seen.
Fig. 85 C: Microfocus magnification view.

Analysis

Form: circumscribed, round
Contours: unsharp; a wide comet tail is directed towards the nipple

Conclusion

Mammographically malignant tumor.
Fig. 85 D: Operative specimen photograph, see Color Plate II.

Histology

8 × 8 mm ductal carcinoma. No axillary metastases.

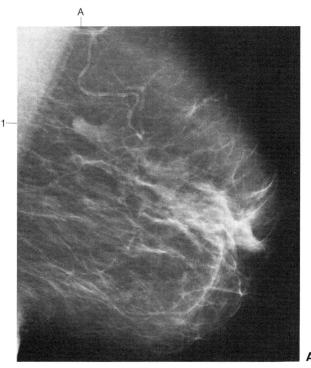

A

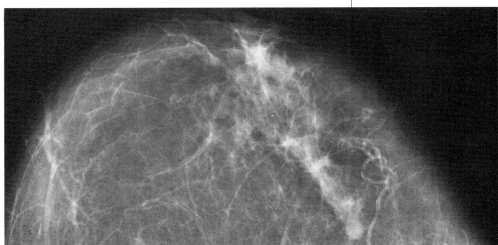

B

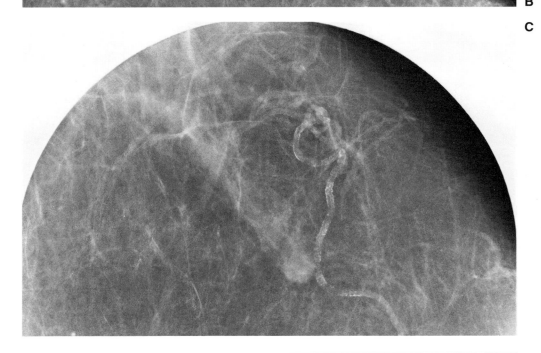

C

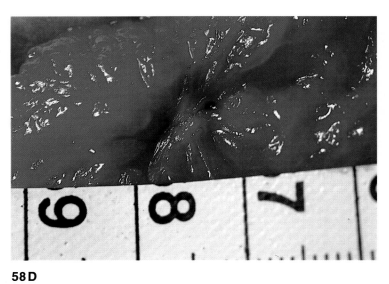

58 D

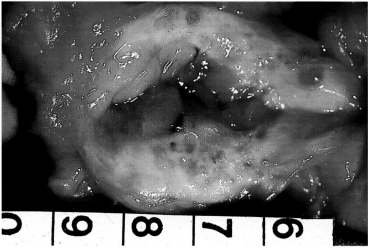

62 C

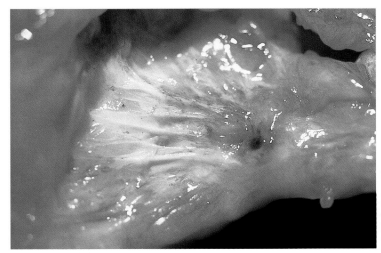

66 B

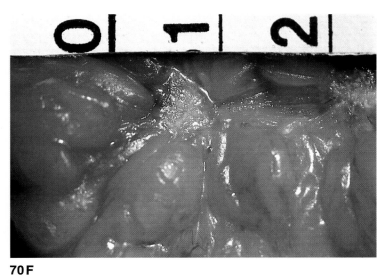

70 F

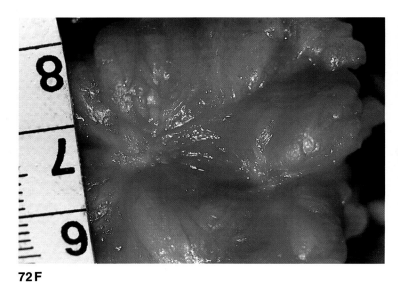

72 F

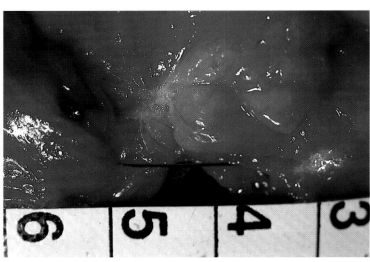

75 E

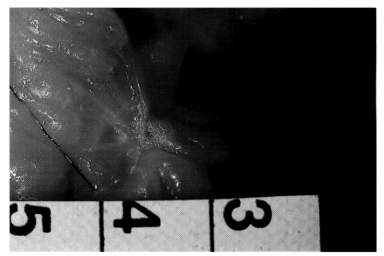

76 F

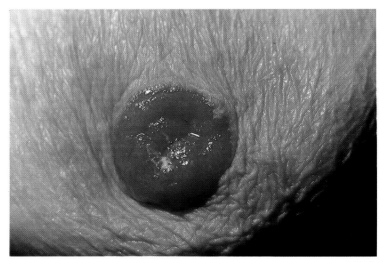

85 D

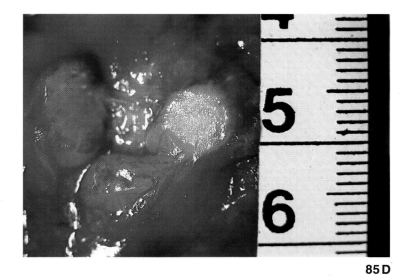

105 A

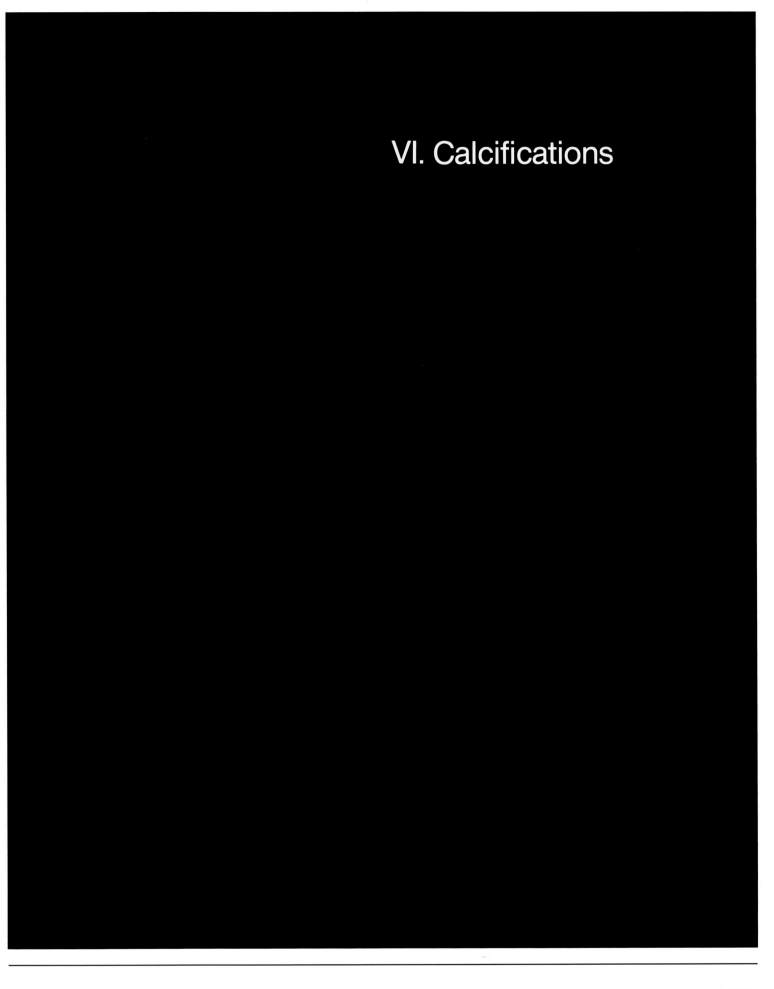

VI. Calcifications

When analyzing calcifications in the absence of a tumor shadow, or if disregarding the tumor shadow, the most important factors are *form, size* and *density* of the individual particles. The *number* and *distribution* of the calcifications should also be taken into consideration.

The *analysis* starts with attempting to discover the pathological process that has produced the calcifications, which assume the shape of the mould into which they have been cast. Therefore, careful analysis of the *form* and *size* of the individual calcifications can lead us to their pathoanatomical location and can indirectly tell us the process that has produced them. Intra- and inter-particulate *density* analysis brings us even closer to understanding the process producing the calcifications.

Most calcifications in the breast are of the benign type. More than 80% of biopsied clusters of calcifications represent benign processes (9, 12).

Detailed analysis of the *form, size* and *density* as well as the *number* and *distribution* of calcifications can lead to a high level of diagnostic accuracy. Microfocus magnification mammography is extremely helpful in many cases since it provides a more detailed image.

The following **terms** are used to simplify the description of calcifications:
- *Cluster:* Distribution of calcifications is restricted to an area on the order of 1 cm².
- *Scattered:* The calcifications are distributed throughout much or most of the breast parenchyma.
- *Casting:* We restrict this term to a configuration frequently seen with intraductal carcinoma, most typically with the comedo type (cases 90, 92, 96, 99, 100, 101, 102, 103, 104, 105, 106, 107, 108, 109).
- *Granular:* Irregular in form, size and density, grouped very close together in an area of the breast. Resembles granulated sugar (cases 86, 87, 88, 94, 95, 98, 107).
- *Punctate:* Very fine, powder-like, often barely perceptible (cases 116, 122, 141).

The key to the analysis of calcifications lies in localizing them to their anatomical site of origin:
- *Ductal:* In terminal ducts and ductules.

- *Lobular:* In cyst-like dilated lobules (see page 170, 171).
- *Miscellaneous:* Arterial wall, periductal, fibroadenoma, sebaceous glands, oil cysts, papilloma, etc. (see page 172).

Ductal-type Calcifications

Proliferation of the ductal epithelium may progress through several stages of atypia to intraductal carcinoma. Concurrent with this process, intraductal calcifications may appear. These may result either from active cellular secretion (1, 12) or from calcification of intraluminal cellular debris (30). Regardless of which of these processes leads to the calcifications, the end results, the so-called malignant-type microcalcifications, are extremely variable in *form, size, density* and *number* (Fig. XVI–XVIII).

Form

Despite their wide variation in appearance, the malignant-type calcifications can be classified into two basic forms:
1) **Granular:** "Calcifications in carcinoma are, generally, tiny, dot-like or somewhat elongated, innumerable and irregularly grouped very close together in an area of the breast, resembling fine grains of salt" (30).
   This description has retained its validity over the years. Much of the irregularity of the individual calcifications may result from the highly irregular nature of the intraductal proliferation producing them (Fig. XVII) (cases 86, 87, 88, 94, 95, 98, 107).
2) **Casting:** These form the most typical and reliable sign of intraductal carcinoma (35, 46) (Fig. XVIII). These are casts of segments of the ductal lumen, sometimes filling in a branch of the duct as well. It is the ductal lumen that determines the maximum width of the castings. The uneven necrosis of the cellular debris and the irregular, active production of the calcification explains the fragmentation and the irregular contour of the castings.

Magnification views reveal that the casting is built of fragments that differ in density, lenght and outline (cases 90, 92, 96, 99–109). Although plasma cell mastitis (periductal mastitis, ductal ectasia) may also produce elongated intraductal calcifications, these have a regular form and outline and a high, uniform density (case 118).

Size

Originally these calcifications lie within the lumen of the duct. With growth and infiltration of the tumor the calcifications become larger through coalescence and tissue necrosis.

Density

When analyzing density one should compare the density of the various parts of the individual calcifications (intraparticulate density analysis) and also compare the densities of the particles with each other (interparticulate density analysis).
Both the granular- and casting-type calcifications show great variations in density within an individual particle and among adjacent particles.

Number

Although the actual number of calcifications has been considered by some to have diagnostic significance, the *form, size* and *density* of the calcifications are of far greater importance. Magnification mammography in particular has demonstrated that the number of calcifications detected can be highly dependent upon the mammography technique. The granular-type calcifications are often innumerable, as one can understand from the pathological background.
It is important to note that the casting-type calcifications are so characteristic of intraductal carcinoma that the diagnosis can be made on the basis of one or two such calcifications alone (cases 101, 105).

Distribution

Intraductal, malignant-type calcifications are usually clustered within an area of the breast, often within one lobe.

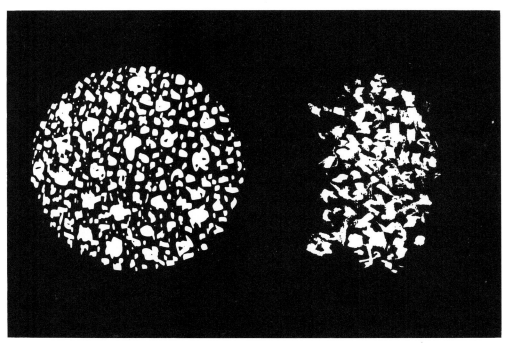

Fig. XVI: Calcifications without an associated tumor: one or more calcifications constitute the entire radiologic abnormality.

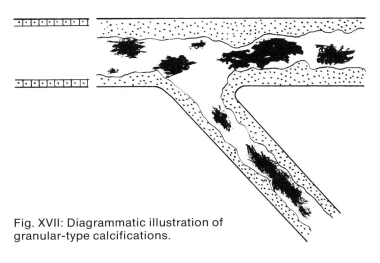

Fig. XVII: Diagrammatic illustration of granular-type calcifications.

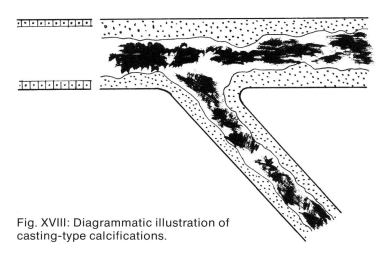

Fig. XVIII: Diagrammatic illustration of casting-type calcifications.

Practice in Calcification Analysis

(Cases 86–109)

86

48-year-old woman, asymptomatic. First screening examination.

Physical Examination

No palpable tumor in the breasts.

Mammography

Fig. 86 A: Right breast, detailed view of the medio-lateral oblique projection. Normal mammogram.
Second screening examination 24 months later. No palpable tumor.
Fig. 86 B: Right breast, detailed view of the medio-lateral oblique projection. A cluster of microcalcifications is now seen in the upper half of the breast (arrow). No associated tumor.
Fig. 86 C & D: Right breast, microfocus magnification views, medio-lateral oblique and cranio-caudal projections.

Analysis of the Calcifications

The tiny, granular, clustered, ductal-type calcifications are irregular in form, size and density. They have arisen since the previous examination. Mammographically malignant-type calcifications.
Fig. 86 E & F: Operative specimen radiographs, magnification view.

Histology

Comedo carcinoma with infiltration. No axillary lymph node metastases.

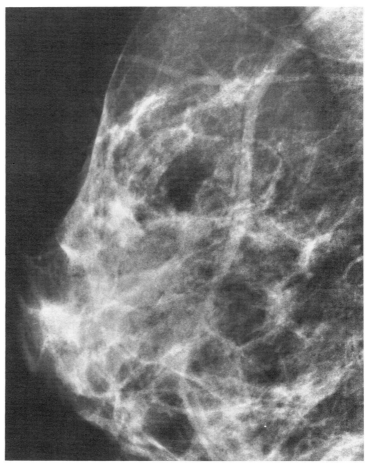

A

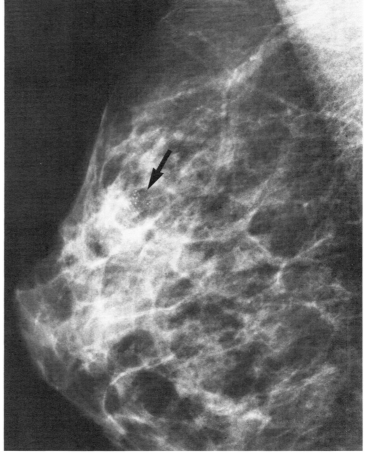

B

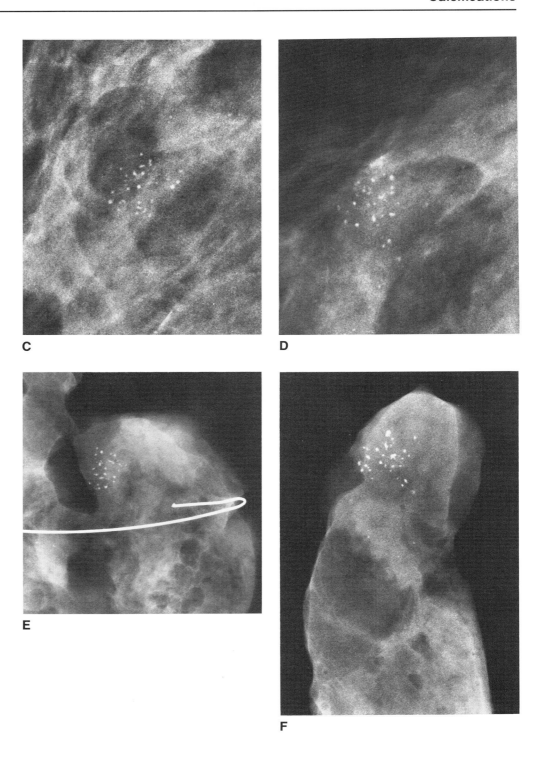

C

D

E

F

87

Asymptomatic 50-year-old woman. First screening study.

Physical Examination

No palpable tumor in the breasts.

Mammography

Fig. 87 A: Left breast, medio-lateral oblique projection. Two clusters of microcalcifications are seen in the upper half of the breast (arrow). In addition, a solitary, 4 mm crescent-shaped calcification is seen in the central portion of the breast, mammographically benign.

Fig. 87 B & C: Magnification view, medio-lateral oblique projection and specimen radiography.

Analysis of the Clustered Calcifications

Form: granular, some elongate; highly irregular

Density: variable

Distribution: cluster, the calcifications are seen very near to each other in a small area of the breast

Conclusion

Mammographically malignant-type (granular) microcalcifications.

Histology

Intraductal carcinoma, non-invasive.

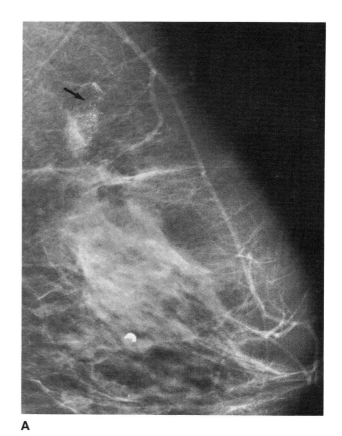

A

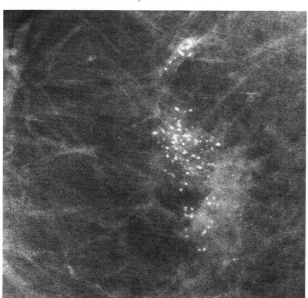

B

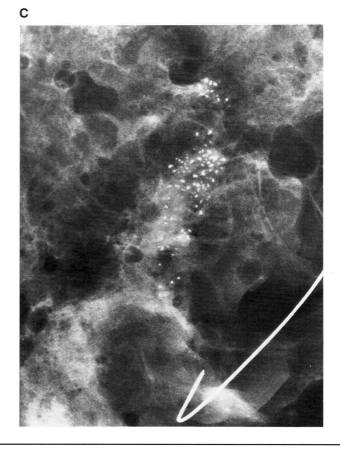

C

88

Fig. 88 A & B: Detailed view of the contact mammogram and microfocus magnification view. Innumerable granular-type calcifications of varying form, size and density. Some calcifications are of the casting type.
Typical mammographic appearance of malignant-type calcifications.

Histology

Infiltrating ductal carcinoma.

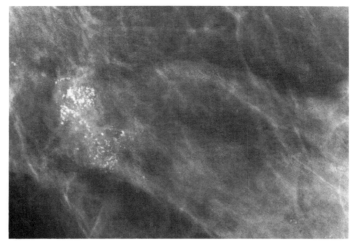

A

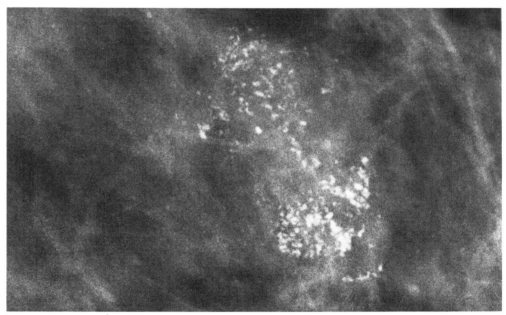

B

89

Fig. 89 A: Right breast, detailed view of the cranio-caudal projection.
Fig. 89 B: Microfocus magnification view.
There are numerous casting-type calcifications indicating the presence of malignancy.

Histology

Multifocal comedo carcinoma, non-infiltrating.

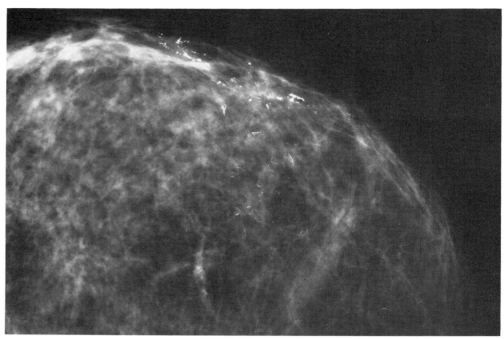

A

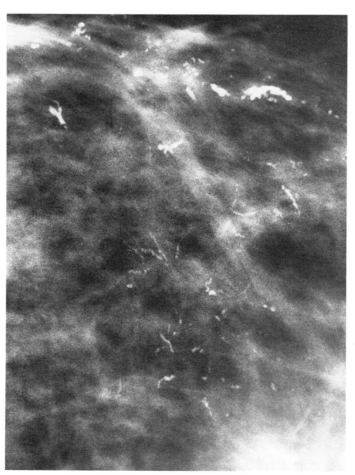

B

90

Fig. 90 A: Detailed view of the medio-lateral oblique projection, left breast. Age 27.

Fig. 90 B: Enlarged view of the calcifications.

There is a cluster of numerous casting-type, branching calcifications, characteristic of carcinoma.

Histology

Infiltrating carcinoma with lymph node metastases.

Comment

Death in two years.

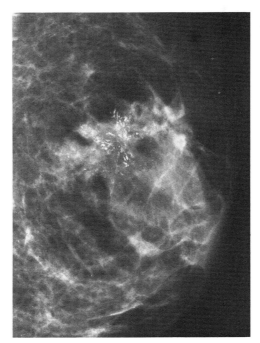

A

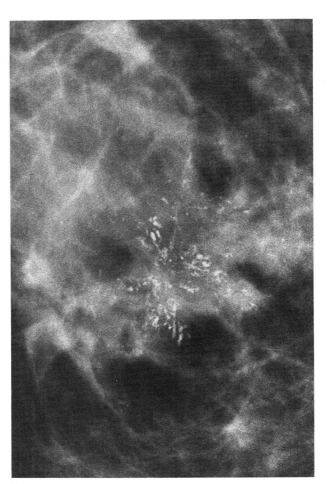

B

91

Fig. 91 A: Right breast, detailed view of the cranio-caudal projection. There are innumerable, clustered, highly irregular, mostly branching, casting-type calcifications of varying size and density. An ill-defined tumor surrounds the calcifications. This may correspond to infiltration.
Fig. 91 B: Microfocus magnification view.

Histology

Infiltrating comedo carcinoma.

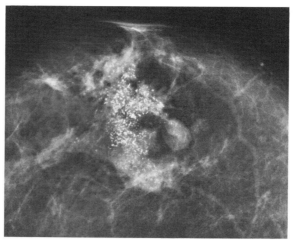

A

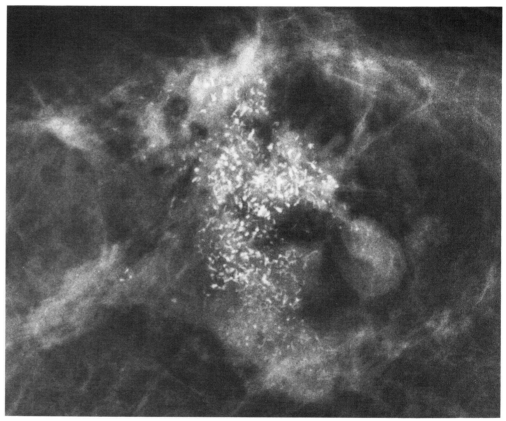

B

92

Fig. 92 A – D: Four examples of malignant type calcifications, mostly casting type.
Magnification reveals that the castings are constructed of fragments that differ in density, width and length and are irregular in outline.

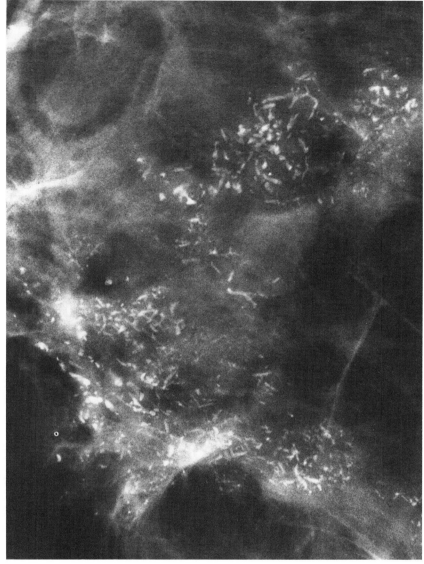

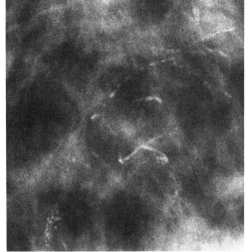

A

B

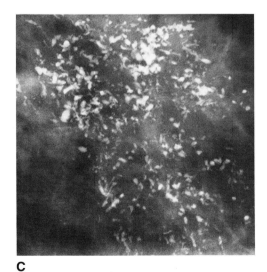

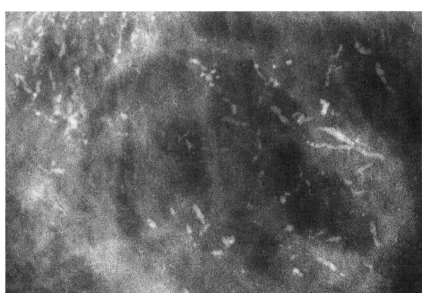

C

D

93

Age 40. Asymptomatic. First screening examination.

Physical Examination

No palpable tumor in the breasts.

Mammography

Fig. 93 A & B: Left breast, detailed views of the medio-lateral oblique and cranio-caudal projections. There is a small group of calcifications in the lower outer quadrant.
Fig. 93 C: Microfocus magnification view of the medio-lateral oblique projection.

Analysis

This is an example of casting-type calcifications. These are formed within segments of a duct and its branches. The ductal lumen contains the irregular epithelial proliferation which gradually undergoes necrosis and becomes partially calcified. There is also an irregular, active production of calcifications, and together these two processes result in the highly variable outline typical of casting-type calcifications. The magnification view reveals that the cast is built of fragments that differ in density, length and outline.
Fig. 93 D: Operative specimen radiograph, magnification.

Histology

Invasive ductal carcinoma. No lymph node metastases.

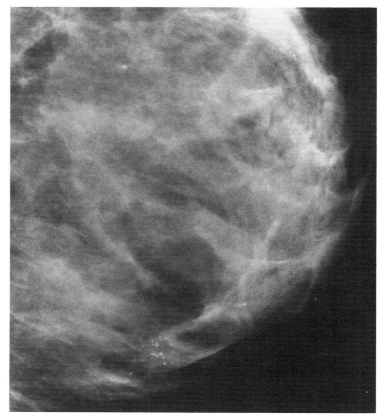

A

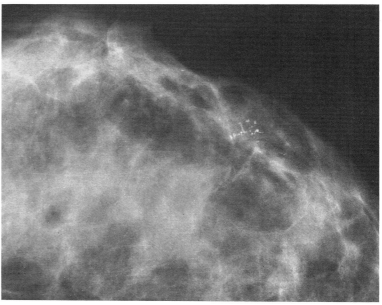

B

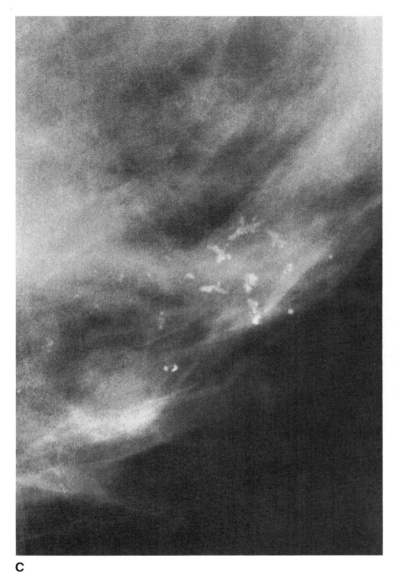

C

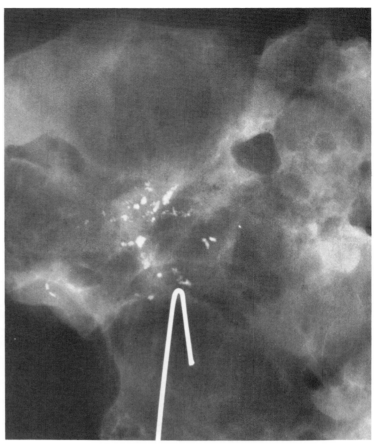

D

94

75-year-old woman, asymptomatic. First screening study.

Physical Examination

No palpable tumor in the breasts.

Mammography

Fig. 94 A & B: Left breast, detailed views of the medio-lateral oblique and cranio-caudal projections. There are two clusters of calcifications within an ill-defined tumor mass in the upper outer quadrant.
Fig. 94 C & D: Microfocus magnification views, medio-lateral oblique and cranio-caudal projections.

Analysis of the Calcifications

Form: highly variable
Density: highly variable, some fade into the background
Distribution: cluster

Conclusion

Mammographically malignant-type calcifications (granular type), within an ill-defined tumor.

Histology

Intraductal carcinoma with minimal invasion.

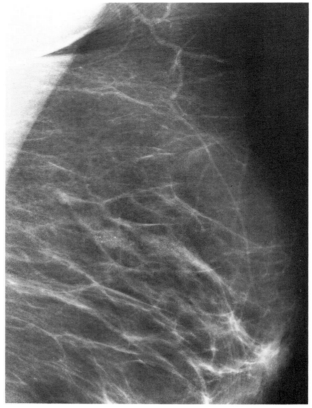

A

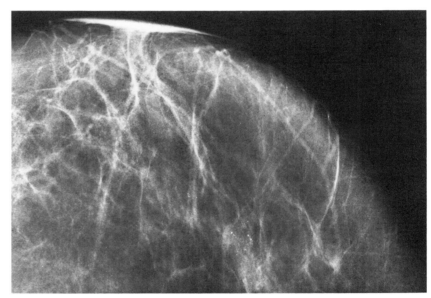

B

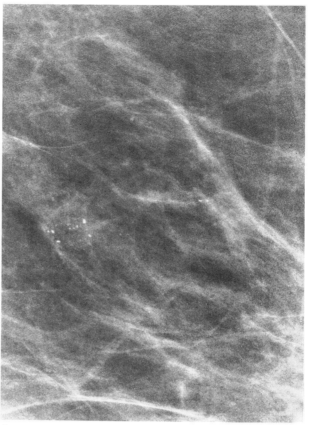

C

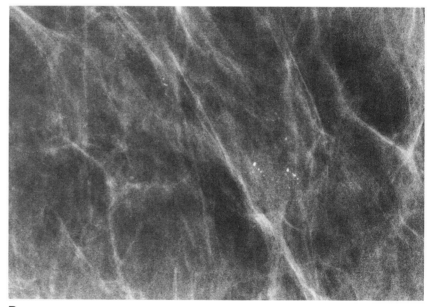

D

95

Age 62, referred for a tumor in the left breast first detected two weeks earlier.

Physical Examination

The palpable tumor is clinically malignant.

Mammography

Fig. 95 A: Left breast, cranio-caudal projection. A cluster of calcifications without a tumor shadow is seen in the lateral half of the breast. A single, oval, smooth-bordered calcification is seen centrally (mammographically benign, liponecrosis microcystica calcificans).
Fig. 95 B: Left breast, microfocus magnification view, cranio-caudal projection.

Analysis of the Clustered Calcifications

Form: highly variable, amorphous, fragmented
Density: variable
Size: highly variable
Distribution: clustered

Conclusion

Typical mammographic appearance of malignant-type calcifications.

Histology

Ductal carcinoma in situ with minimal infiltration.

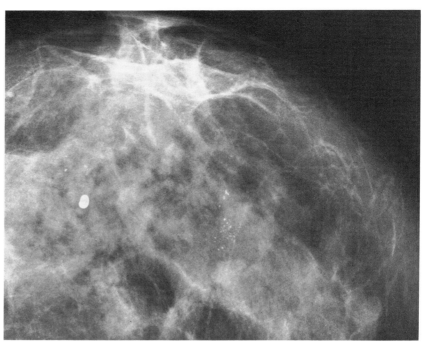

A

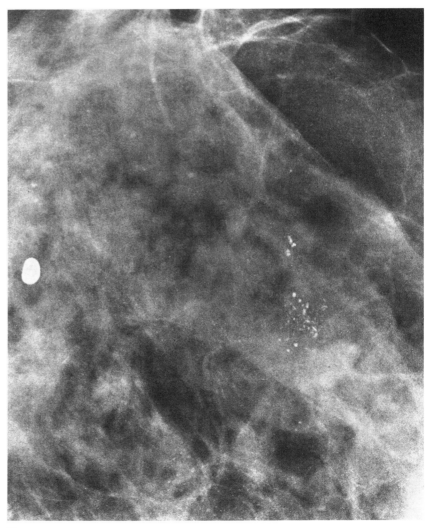

B

96

Age 61, asymptomatic. First screening study.

Physical Examination

No palpable tumor in the breasts.

Mammography

Fig. 96 A: Right breast, medio-lateral oblique projection. A cluster of calcifications is seen in the axillary portion of the breast (arrow). No associated tumor.
Fig. 96 B: Right breast, microfocus magnification view, medio-lateral oblique projection.

Analysis

Form: granular and casting type
Density: highly variable
Size: small, although considerable variation
Distribution: cluster

Conclusion

Mammographically malignant-type calcifications.

Histology

Intraductal carcinoma in situ.

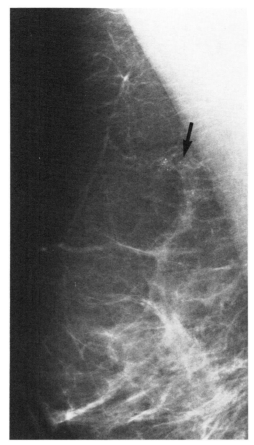

A

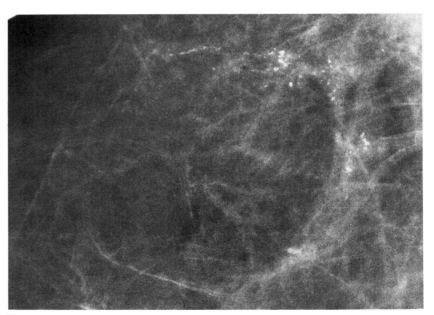

B

97

48-year-old woman, referred for an abscess in the right breast. No palpable tumor in the left breast.

Mammography

Fig. 97 A: *Left* breast, detailed view of the cranio-caudal projection. Mammographically benign tumor (open arrows) in the lateral portion of the breast. Immediately superficial to the tumor a cluster of calcifications is seen (solid arrow).

Fig. 97 B: *Left* breast, microfocus magnification view, cranio-caudal projection. The cluster of calcifications (solid arrow) is more clearly seen. In addition, numerous scattered calcifications are revealed.

Fig. 97 C: *Left* breast, operative specimen radiograph, magnification view.

Analysis of the Calcifications in the Left Breast

The clustered calcifications are irregular in form, density and size. They are a mixture of granular and casting types, mammographically highly suspicious for malignancy. Many of the scattered calcifications are of the lobular type.

Fig. 97 D: *Right* breast, detailed view in the medio-lateral oblique projection, lower portion of the breast.

Fig. 97 E: Operative specimen radiograph with microfocus magnification.

Analysis of the Calcifications in the Right Breast

Form: lobular type, round, sharply outlined
Density: fairly uniform
Distribution: scattered

Conclusion, Right Breast

Mammographically benign-type calcifications (lobular type).

Histology

Left breast: Carcinoma in situ. Sclerosing adenosis, atypical lobular hyperplasia.
Right breast: Sclerosing adenosis, blunt duct adenosis. No epithelial proliferation or atypia.

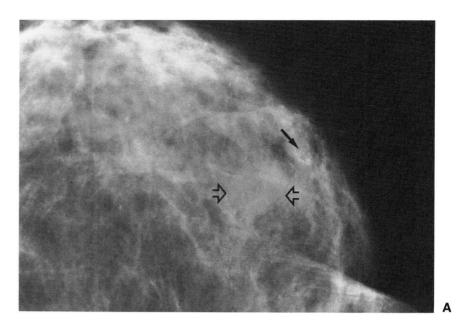

A

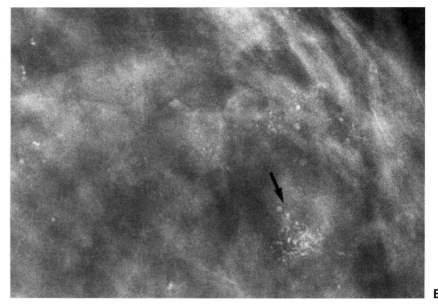

B

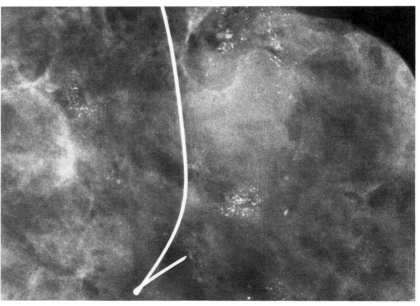

C

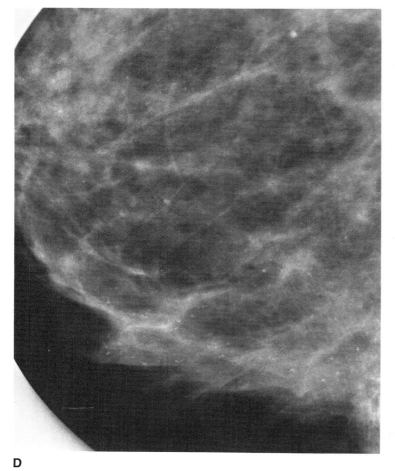

D

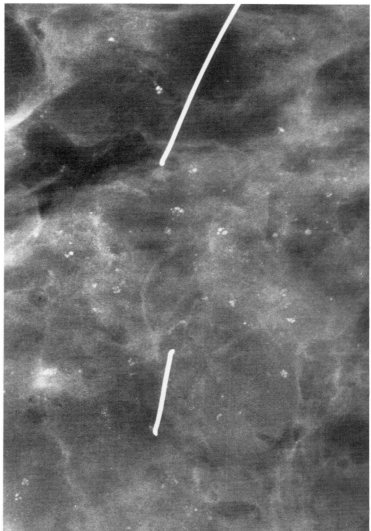

E

98

67-year-old woman, asymptomatic. First screening study.

Physical Examination

No palpable tumor in the breasts.

Mammography

Fig. 98 A: Left breast, detailed view of the cranio-caudal projection. A few small calcifications are demonstrated (arrows).
Fig. 98 B: Enlarged coned-down compression view, cranio-caudal projection.
Fig. 98 C: Microfocus magnification view, cranio-caudal projection. The cluster of calcifications is seen adjacent to a partially calcified artery.

Analysis

The clustered calcifications are of the ductal type. Some are granular, some elongated. They vary considerably in shape and density and are of different sizes.

Conclusion

Mammographically malignant-type calcifications.

Histology

Intraductal carcinoma in situ.

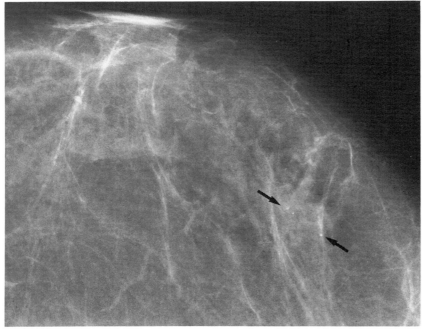

A

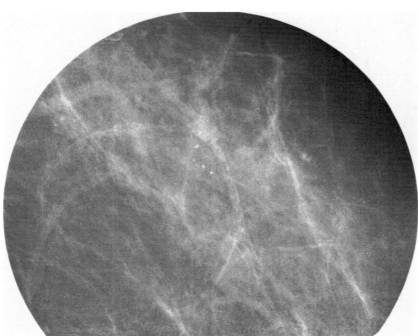

B

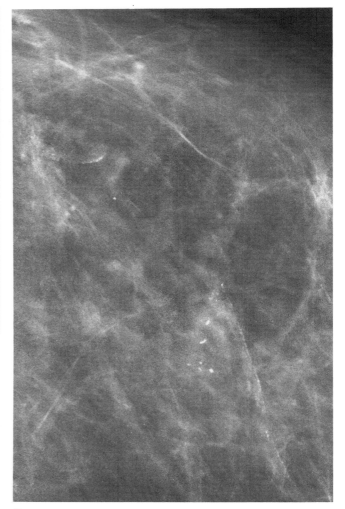

C

99

74-year-old woman, not aware of any breast abnormality. First screening examination.

Mammography

Fig. 99 A: Left breast, detailed view of the medio-lateral oblique projection. In the upper outer quadrant there is a 5 × 5 cm area containing numerous calcifications associated with an ill-defined density.

Fig. 99 B & C: Microfocus magnification views, medio-lateral oblique and cranio-caudal projections. Most of the calcifications are of the casting type, typical of ductal carcinoma.

Analysis

This case gives an excellent opportunity to anlyze these calcifications. The shape of the cast is determined by the uneven, active production of calcification and the irregular necrosis of the cellular debris. The contours of the cast are always irregular and the cast is always fragmented. Density analysis reveals that within one cast the several fragments may differ in density. The cast may be branched.

Histology

Poorly differentiated ductal carcinoma with stromal infiltration.

Note:

The infiltration probably accounts for some of the density surrounding the calcifications.

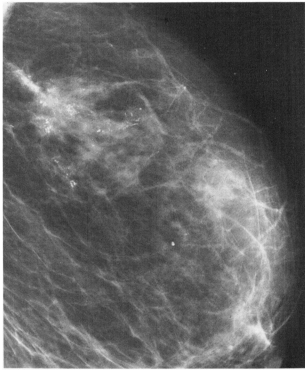

A

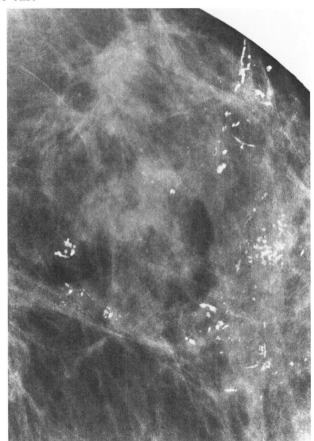

C

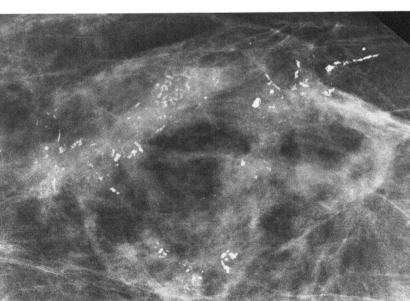

B

100

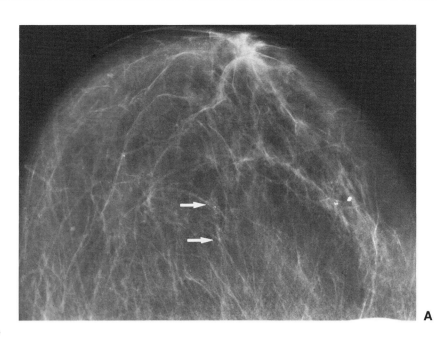

Fig. 100 A: Left breast, cranio-caudal projection. There is a cluster of calcifications, centrally located (arrows).
Fig. 100 B: Microfocus magnification view of the microcalcifications, cranio-caudal projection.

Analysis

Typical intraductal, casting-type calcifications. They are irregular in shape, size and density, and follow the course of a duct and its branches.

Conclusion

Mammographically malignant-type calcifications.

Histology

Non-invasive intraductal carcinoma.

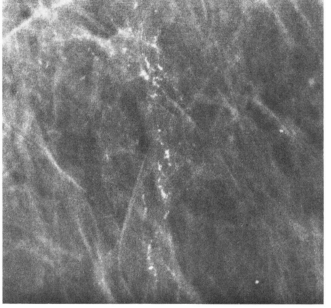

101

Fig. 101 A: Right breast, cranio-caudal projection. Typical casting-type calcifications (solid arrow). There is also a single, larger, homogenous, linear calcification with smooth borders, characteristic of plasma cell mastitis (open arrow).

Fig. 101 B: Coned-down compression view, cranio-caudal projection. The typical casting-type calcifications, one of them branching, are mammographic signs of carcinoma.

Histology

Intraductal carcinoma in situ.

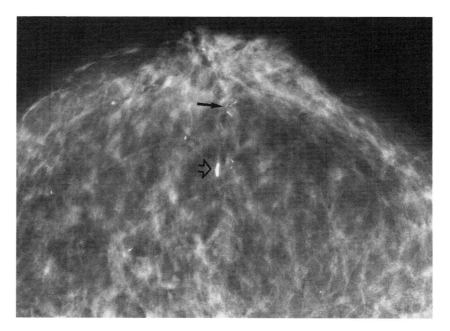

B

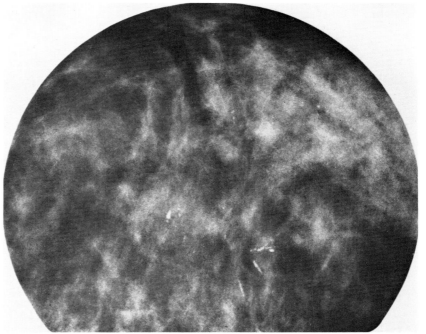

102

28-year-old woman, felt a lump in the upper outer quadrant of the right breast.

Physical Examination

No distinct tumor mass but the entire upper outer quadrant of the right breast was hard and there was a large axillary lymph node.

Mammography

Fig. 102 A, B, C: Right breast, detailed views of the medio-lateral oblique projection with contact (A) and microfocus magnification mammography (B & C). The entire upper half of the breast is filled with innumerable calcifications. Most striking, one duct and its main branches are completely filled with calcifications all the way to the nipple. No associated tumor.

Fig. 102 D: Operative specimen magnification radiograph.

Analysis

An unusual picture of innumerable casting-type calcifications spread over a large area of the breast.

Conclusion

Typical appearance of malignant-type calcifications.

Histology

Intraductal and infiltrative comedo carcinoma over an area of at least 15 cm diameter. Axillary lymph node metastases.

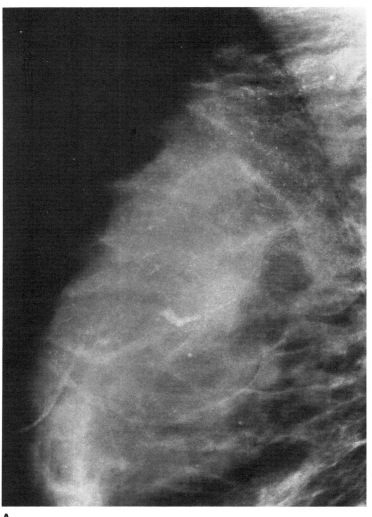

A

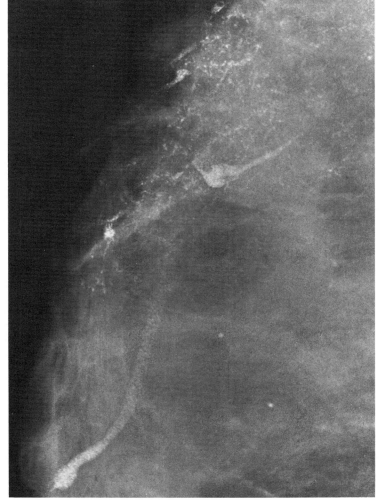

B

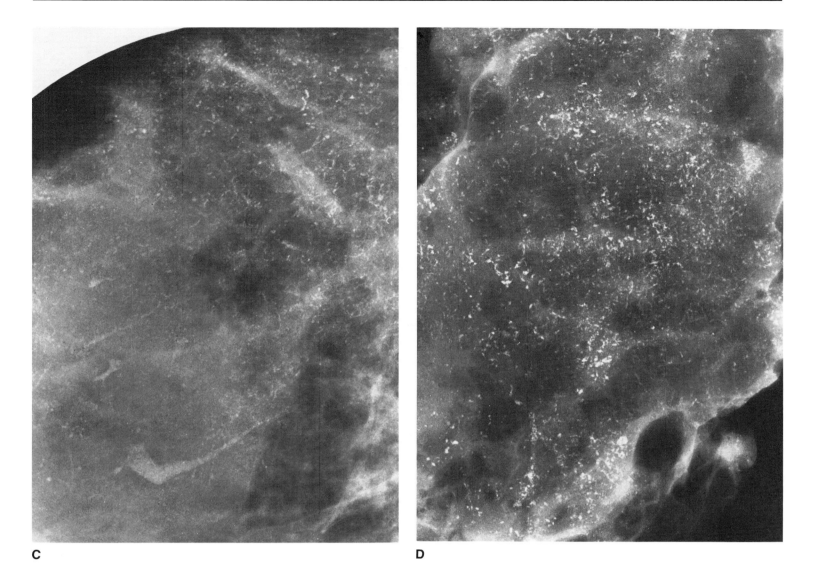

C

D

103

62-year-old woman, asymptomatic.
First screening study.

Physical Examination

No palpable tumor in the breasts.

Mammography

Fig. 103 A: Left breast, detailed view
of the cranio-caudal and medio-lateral
projection. A circumscribed tumor
with associated calcifications is seen
5 cm from the nipple.

Analysis of the Tumor

Form: circumscribed, oval, lobulated
Contour: partly sharply outlined; seg-
ments of a halo sign are seen in
Fig. 103 B & C (arrows); parenchymal
structures obscure part of the tumor
border
Density: low density radiopaque
Size: 15 × 10 mm

Conclusion

Mammographically benign tumor.

Analysis of the Calcifications

Form: highly irregular, some of them
casting type
Density: highly variable
Distribution: within the tumor

Conclusion

Mammographically malignant type
calcifications.

Comment

Mammographically the tumor is
benign (probably fibroadenoma), but
the calcifications are of the malignant
type. Cancer within a fibroadenoma,
however rare, is the logical diagnostic
choice.

Histology

Carcinoma within a fibroadenoma.

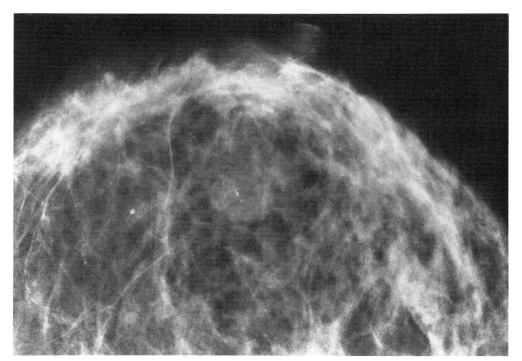

A

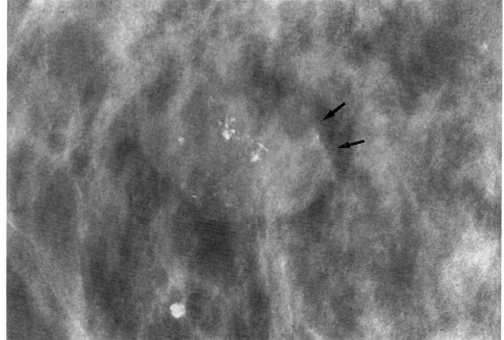

B

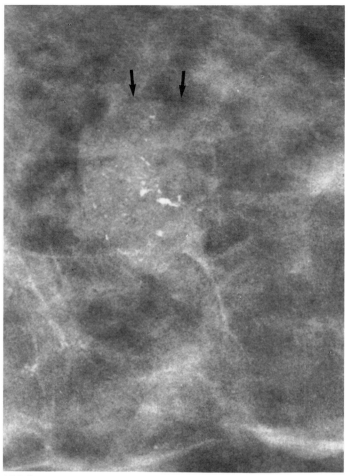

103 C

104

Fig. 104: Left breast, microfocus magnification view in the medio-lateral oblique projection. Numerous calcifications are seen, with no associated tumor.

Analysis

Typical casting-type calcifications. These are mammographically characteristic of malignancy. A single, dense, benign-type periductal calcification (arrow) is superimposed.

Histology

Intraductal carcinoma with minimal invasion. No axillary lymph node metastases.

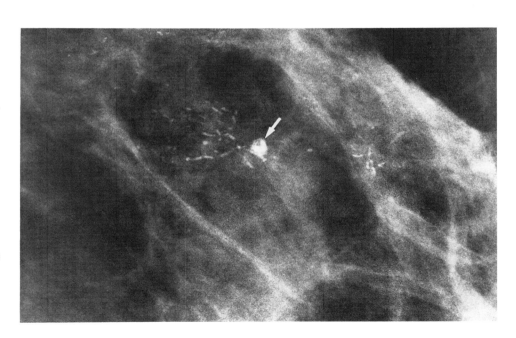

105

Age 80, two month history of eczematous change of the nipple.

Physical Examination

Fig. 105 A: The appearance of the nipple resembles Paget's disease. No palpable breast tumor.

Mammography

Fig. 105 B: Left breast, microfocus magnification view, medio-lateral oblique projection. A single casting type calcification (solid arrow) and a group of granular type calcifications (open arrow) are seen with no associated tumor. An additional solitary, benign type, smooth bordered calcification is readily apparent (liponecrosis microcystica calcificans).

Analysis

Both the granular- and casting-type calcifications indicate the presence of a malignant lesion.

Conclusion

One has to search for the carcinoma focus in a patient with Paget's disease. The described malignant-type calcifications indicate the site of an intraductal carcinoma.

Histology

Non-invasive intraductal carcinoma. Paget's disease of the breast.

Comment

Paget's disease of the breast, first described by J. Paget in 1874, is a special form of ductal carcinoma associated with eczematous changes of the nipple. The clinical picture is dominated by the malignant nipple lesion, and the ductal carcinoma is usually occult to palpation. Mammography can lead to the detection of the ductal carcinoma in most cases.

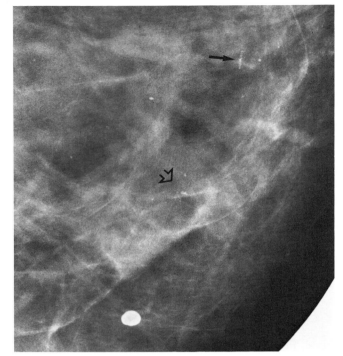

B

Fig. 105 A see Color Plate II, after p. 136.

106

47-year-old woman, asymptomatic.
First screening study.

Mammography

Fig. 106 A: Right breast, medio-lateral oblique projection. No mammographic abnormality.
Second screening study two years later. The patient is asymptomatic, no palpable tumor in the breasts at physical examination.
Fig. 106 B: Right breast, medio-lateral oblique projection. Small cluster of calcifications 4 cm from the nipple. No associated tumor.
Fig. 106 C & D: Right breast, micro-focus magnification view of the calcifications.

Analysis

Form: irregular, some casting-type calcifications, some amorphous and fragmented
Density: variable
Distribution: cluster

Conclusion

Newly arising, mammographically malignant-type calcifications.

Histology

Comedo carcinoma with minimal infiltration.

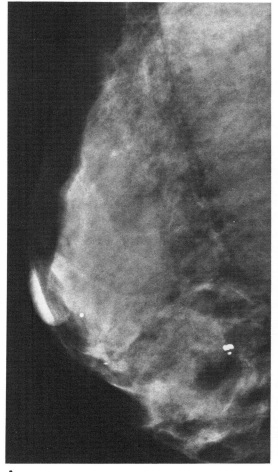

A

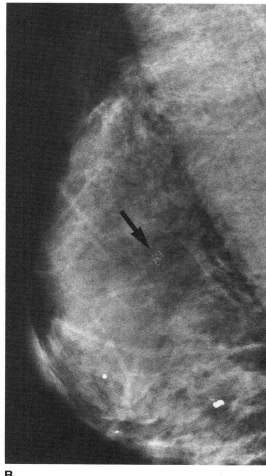

B

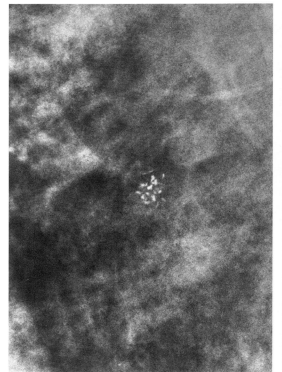

C

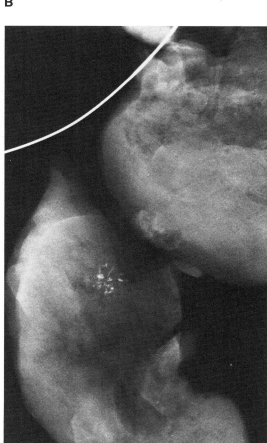

D

107

47-year-old woman with a self-detected tumor in the upper outer quadrant of the right breast.

Physical Examination

The tumor appears malignant and there are enlarged axillary lymph nodes.

Mammography

Fig. 107 A: Right breast, medio-lateral oblique projection. Dense breast with scattered calcifications throughout the breast. No associated tumor shadow.
Fig. 107 B & C: Right breast, medio-lateral oblique projection, microfocus magnification views of the upper (B) and lower (C) halves of the breast.

Analysis (best on the magnification views)

Form: highly irregular, partly granular and elongated, some branching in the lower half of the breast
Density: highly variable
Distribution: many clusters distributed throughout the breast

Conclusion

The granular- and casting-type calcifications are of the mammographically malignant type, spread throughout the parenchyma, suggesting a multicentric carcinoma. There is a small cluster of highly dense, sharply outlined oval calcifications in the lower half of the breast that are of the mammographically benign type.

Histology

Poorly differentiated, multicentric, infiltrative ductal carcinoma. Axillary metastases with periglandular growth.

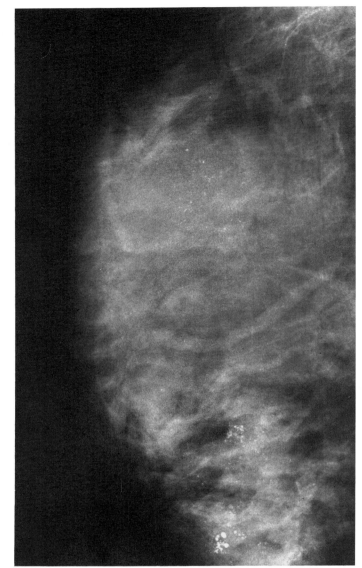

A

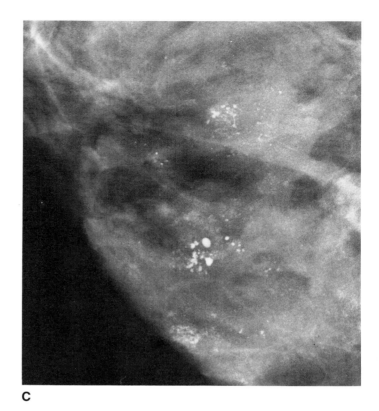

C

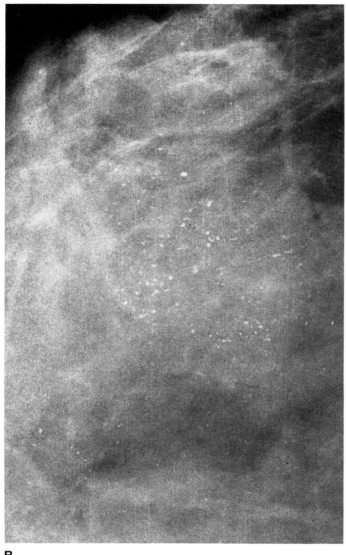

B

108

43-year-old woman referred for a recently detected lump in the upper outer quadrant of the right breast. The tumor was clinically suspicious for malignancy.

Mammography

Fig. 108 A & B: Right breast, medio-lateral oblique projection, contact and microfocus magnification. A cluster of calcifications is seen associated with a tumor. This tumor can hardly be differentiated from the dense, homogenous parenchyma.

Analysis of the Calcifications

Form: irregular, a mixture of granular- and casting-type calcifications
Size: highly variable
Density: highly variable
Distribution: cluster

Conclusion

Mammographically typical picture of malignant-type (granular and casting) calcifications.

Histology

Infiltrative comedo carcinoma with axillary lymph node metastases.

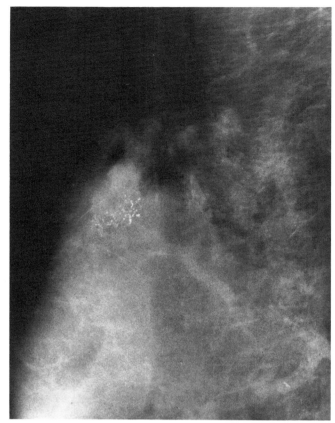

A

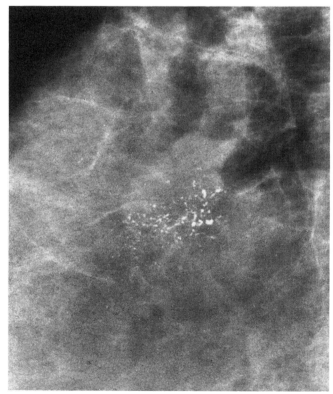

B

109

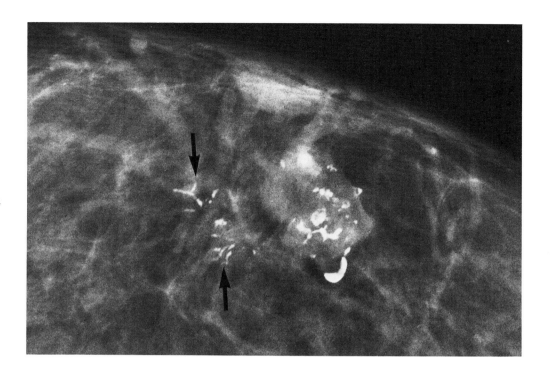

77-year-old asymptomatic woman. First screening study.

Mammography

Fig. 109: Detail of the cranio-caudal projection. Microfocus magnification of the retroareolar region. There is a retroareolar tumor with coarse associated calcifications.
One cm medial to the tumor there is a small cluster of calcifications without a tumor shadow (arrows).

Analysis of the Tumor

Form: circumscribed, lobulated
Contour: no halo sign, unsharp contour
Density: low density radiopaque

Analysis of the Intratumoral Calcifications

Form: irregular, coarse
Size: variable
Density: high
Distribution: within and immediately adjacent to the tumor

Conclusion

Mammographically benign-type calcifications within a tumor of low density. Most probably a calcified fibroadenoma.

Analysis of the Calcifications Adjacent to the Tumor

Form: irregular, branched, elongated, fragmented
Density: variable within the same elongated calcification

Conclusion

Casting-type calcifications, typical for ductal carcinoma.

Histology

Partially calcified fibroadenoma. The casting-type calcifications were associated with infiltrative ductal carcinoma.

Lobular-type Calcifications

Normal lobules demonstrated by galactography in Fig. 110. *Pathological* dilatation of ductules and whole lobules is demonstrated by galactography in Fig. 111, illustrating the sites where these calcifications may arise. The differentiation among the separate pathological entities leading to calcification within the lobules (sclerosing adenosis, atypical lobular hyperplasia, cystic hyperplasia, blunt duct adenosis) is the task of the pathologist.

When the calcifications can be localized to the dilated lobules on the basis of their *form, size, density* and *distribution,* the above-mentioned histopathological processes should be considered, cystic hyperplasia in particular.

Form

These calcifications arise within a spherical cavity that determines their form. The entire contents of the cavity may calcify, producing a *homogenous, solid, sharply outlined, spherical, pearl-like density* (Fig. XIX B & C) (cases 112, 113, 115, 116, 121).

The smaller the cavity, the more likely the contents are to calcify completely. This is the typical picture of sclerosing adenosis (Fig. XIX D) (cases 119, 121).

In cystic hyperplasia, when the lobular dilatation results in somewhat larger cavities, the cystic fluid may contain freely mobile particles, "milk of calcium", which settle to the dependent portion of the cavities. These are seen on the lateral view as crescent-shaped or elongate calcifications, which may resemble a teacup seen from the side (Fig. XIX E & F) (Ref. 25). On the cranio-caudal view these calcifications are circular, faint, opaque smudges, resembling a teacup seen from above (Ref. 53).

Size

The more the surrounding fibrosis compresses the lobules the smaller the intra-ductular calcifications are. These small, punctate calcifications with surrounding homogenous fibrosis are typical of cystic hyperplasia and sclerosing

adenosis. There tends to be little variation in size among the calcifications. In cystic hyperplasia the variable saccular dilatation of the lobules (Fig. 111) produces moulds of differing sizes. The larger the cavity the less likely it is to become completely calcified (cases 113, 114, 120).

Density

Small, pearl-like calcifications are uniform and dense. *Calcifications in larger, saccular* cavities differ somewhat in density according to size.

Number and distribution

The lobular-type calcifications may be numerous and scattered throughout much of the breast parenchyma.

Comment

Cystic hyperplasia may rarely be associated with lobular carcinoma *in situ.* However, most cases have been incidental findings at serial histological sectioning, located at some distance from the calcifications. Diagnosis of lobular carcinoma in situ cannot be reliably made by mammography.

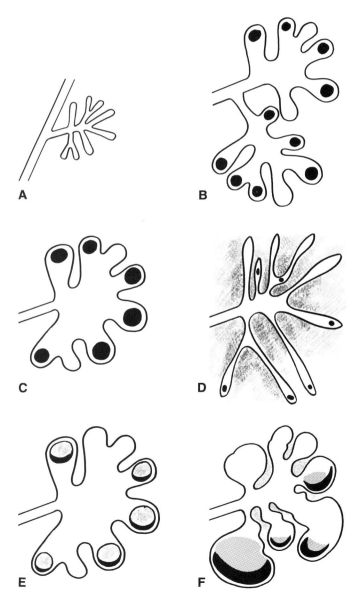

Fig. XIX A−F: Lobular-type calcifications.
A: normal lobule,
B & C: adenosis,
D: sclerosing adenosis,
E & F: cystic hyperplasia.

110
111

In these cases the pathological duct system is demonstrated in one lobe with the help of ductography.
Normal Lobules: Fig. 110, marked "A".
Pathologically dilated, saccular, spherical lobules: Fig. 110, marked "B" and "C", as well as Fig. 111.
The cyst-like dilatations contain stagnating fluid which eventually calcifies. The calcifications arise within spherical cavities that determine their form:
1) When the entire contents of the cavity calcify, the result is numerous spherical and oval, homogenous, smooth-bordered and sharply outlined calcifications, sometimes lobulated or septate (when large), scattered within one or more lobes (case 112).
   The smaller the cavity the more likely the contents are to calcify completely.
   This picture is seen in
   — Sclerosing adenosis: *small, punctate, uniform calcifications* (cases 119, 121).
   — Cystic hyperplasia: *often contains larger, lobulated or septate calcifications* (cases 112, 113, 115, 116).
   — Atypical lobular hyperplasia: *there may be a wide variation in form and size among the calcifications* (case 126).
2) When the calcifications settle to the dependent portion of the cystic dilatations, the result is eccentric, crescent-shaped, teacup-like, scattered calcifications (cases 113, 114, 120).

Conclusion

When the mammogram shows considerable fibrosis and scattered calcifications that are spherical, oval or teacup-shaped with little variation in form, size and density, such calcifications have almost certainly been produced by cystic hyperplasia. Sclerosing

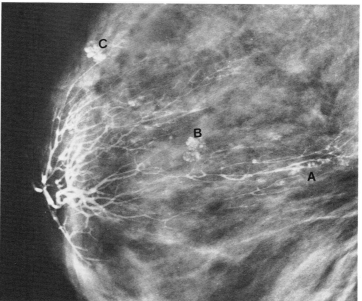

110

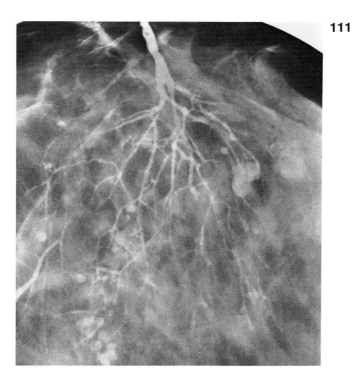

111

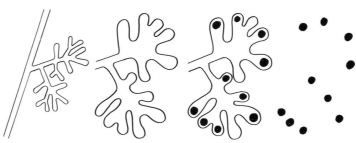

Fig. XX: Involutional-type calcifications. These may result from a mild degree of cystic hyperplasia that calcifies during involution. The glandular tissue atrophies, leaving behind the calcifications within one or more lobes.

adenosis, blunt duct adenosis, atypical lobular hyperplasia (case 126) or very rarely lobular carcinoma in situ may be revealed by histology.

Involutional Type Calcifications

These are mostly seen against a fatty background. They may result from a mild degree of cystic hyperplasia which calcifies during involution. The glandular tissue undergoes atrophy, leaving behind the very fine, punctate calcifications within one or more lobes (Fig. XX, cases 116, 122, 141).

Miscellaneous Calcifications

Arterial Calcifications

Arterial calcifications are usually easy to recognize because the calcified arterial walls have a typical radiologic appearance. When calcification is sparse it may be difficult to recognize the arterial origin of these intermittent calcifications.

Periductal mastitis

(Ductal Ectasia, Plasma Cell Mastitis)

Periductal mastitis produces a typical mammographic appearance. This condition results from extravasation of intraductal secretions causing a periductal chemical mastitis. This sterile, inflammatory reaction is characterized by the presence of plasma cells surrounding the dilated duct. Periductal fibrosis and intraductal and/or periductal calcifications are the final results.
The calcifications can be located
- around the dilated ducts (most frequently),
- inside the lumen or
- in the duct wall.

Form

a) **Periductal** (cases 117, 125):
  - A calcified ring lies within the fibrous tissue which surrounds the dilated duct. The lumen of the duct is well seen inside the calcified ring.

  - When the calcification extends around and along the duct, it appears oval or elongated. Fibrosis accompanies these hollow calcifications.

b) **Intraductal** (cases 118, 123): The secretion inside the duct may calcify, filling in segments of the duct with fairly uniform linear, often needle-like, occasionally branching calcifications of varying length and width.

Density

a) **Periductal:** Both ring or elongate forms have a center of varying lucency, corresponding to the lumen of the duct. The periphery of the calcifications is very dense.
b) **Intraductal:** High, uniform density.

Number and Distribution

Multiple, often bilateral, scattered, oriented towards the nipple, following the course of the ducts.

Comment

Differentiation of the benign intraductal calcifications of plasma cell mastitis from the malignant type casting calcifications of intraductal carcinoma can be easily done as the benign type have a high and uniform density, a generally wide caliber, and tend to follow the course of the normal ducts (maintain a polarity directed toward the nipple).

Sebaceous Gland Calcifications

These are easily recognized and should never lead to confusion (case 124).

Form

Ring-shaped, oval.

Size

Same as skin pores.

Density

The center is always radiolucent.

Number and Distribution

Often very numerous. Occur only within the skin.

Small, Ring-like Calcifications

These may be caused by fat necrosis, called liponecrosis microcystica calcificans (28). They are calcified microhematomas (cases 129, 133).

Form

The calcified surface of the spherical hematoma looks like a small eggshell.

Size

Up to a few mm in diameter.

Density

High and uniform in the periphery, lucent and often irregular at the center. No associated fibrosis.

Number and Distribution

Ranges from solitary to numerous. Usually subcutaneous but may occur anywhere in the breast.

Larger Eggshell-like Calcifications

These are caused by hemorrhage within a spherical or ovoid pathological lesion. The extravasated blood eventually leads to a shell-like calcification. The following pathological entities come under consideration:
a) **Oil cysts** (cases 4, 134, 135, 139) are almost invariably a result of surgery. Fat decomposes to liquid fatty acids that collect at the site of surgical incision. A fibrotic capsule surrounds these oily collections. The fatty acids precipitate as calcium soaps at this capsular surface, eventually forming a thin layer of calcification surrounding the oil cyst (liponecrosis macrocystica calcificans).
Form: Spherical or oval.
Size: Variable, up to several cm.
Density: The lesion has an eggshell-like calcification but the oily content is radiolucent. This characteristic appearance makes the mammographic picture unmistakable.
b) **A larger cyst with eggshell-like calcification** is a rare finding (cases 136, 137). Although eggshell-like

calcifications are almost invariably benign, the rare exception is a smaller retroareolar eggshell-like calcification. This may represent an intraductal, intracystic papilloma or intracystic carcinoma (case 137).

c) **Fibroadenoma** with eggshell-like calcification is rare. This has a center of parenchymal density while the oil cyst has a radiolucent center. The calcification also differs from that seen in cysts or oil cysts.

Papilloma, Papillomatosis

These rarely calcify. The appearance is usually typical (cases 127, 128, 130, 131, 132).

Form

Configuration similar to a raspberry.

Size

Limited to the size of a dilated duct.

Density

High, may be uniform but often contain small, oval-shaped lucent areas.

Number and Distribution

Solitary, tend to be central or retroareolar. In papillomatosis these are located in a main duct and its branches (case 127).

Fibroadenomas

Fibroadenomas may present with three different types of calcification:
1) Coarse, irregular but sharply outlined, very dense calcification. This bizarre appearance is diagnostic of an old fibroadenoma which has undergone myxoid degeneration. The calcification may involve part or all of the fibroadenoma (cases 142, 143, 144).
2) Peripheral calcification in a fibroadenoma may take the appearance of an eggshell (case 138), or may be flecked (cases 145, 146, 147, 148, 149).
The density of these calcifications is high and uniform. Their size and shape may vary; the smaller the

size, the more difficult the differentiation from malignant-type calcifications.
3) Carcinoma within a fibroadenoma: If a benign tumor contains malignant-type calcifications, of either the granular or casting type, malignancy should be suspected (case 103).

Hemangiomas

Hemangiomas (cases 23, 151) may present with either small calcifications that vary in form and size or with larger, bizarre calcifications.

Warts

Warts may rarely calcify. Those that do may be deceptive on the mammogram (case 152).

Strategy

Ductal-type calcifications (granular and casting) represent a malignant process and should be biopsied whether or not there is a palpable lesion.
Miscellaneous calcifications seldom cause differential diagnostic problems and should not be biopsied when the appearance is typical (of fat necrosis, plasma cell mastitis, hyalinizing fibroadenoma, arterial calcifications, sebaceous gland calcifications, etc.). Although **lobular-type calcifications** do not represent a malignant process, they may occasionally resemble the ductal-type calcifications and cause problems in differential diagnosis. In this situation biopsy is necessary.

Practice in Calcification Analysis

(Cases 112–152)

112

43-year-old woman with pain in the breasts and grayish secretion from several ducts of the right breast.

Mammography

Fig. 112: Right breast, detailed view of the cranio-caudal projection (micro-focus magnification view).
Homogeneous fibrosis with numerous lobular-type calcifications of varying size, scattered within the fibrous tissue.

Note

Compare with cases 110 and 111 where the dilated lobules are demonstrated on galactograms.

Analysis of the Calcifications

Form: spherical, some lobulated; the largest calcifications have a septated structure; these are lobular-type calcifications, situated in terminal, cyst-like dilated ductules. Those cyst-like dilatations that are only partially calcified present as faint smudges because they are imaged **en face** with a vertical beam. The same calcifications appear crescentic (teacup-shaped) when imaged with a horizontal beam.
Size: variable
Density: faint, uniform
Distribution: scattered

Conclusion

Extensive fibrosis with lobular-type calcifications is typical of cystic hyperplasia.

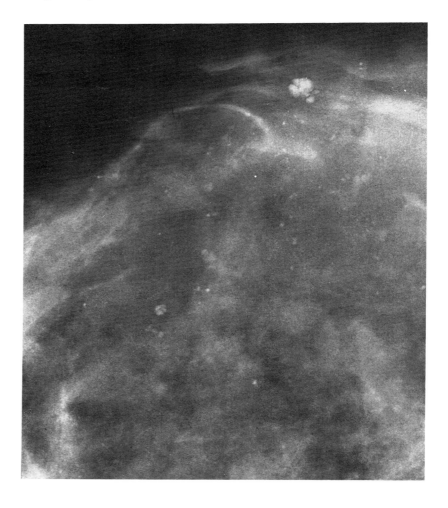

113

52-year-old woman, first screening study. Previous biopsy of the right breast. No palpable tumor.

Mammography

Fig. 113 A: Right breast, medio-lateral oblique projection. There is an extensive fibrosis over much of the breast, with numerous calcifications. No tumor is seen.

Fig. 113 B: Microfocus magnification view, medio-lateral oblique projection. There are three different kinds of calcifications.

Analysis best on the magnification view)

1) The linear calcifications (solid arrows) correspond to the site of operation. They are smooth-bordered and highly dense and appear to be benign, possibly the consequence of postoperative traumatic fat necrosis.

2) The punctate calcifications (open arrow) are small, round and sharply outlined, with uniform density. These are lobular-type, mammographically benign.

3) There are several larger, spherical and oval, partially calcified, cyst-like lesions (dilated lobules). The calcifications themselves are crescent like, teacup-shaped and situated in the dependent, caudal portions of the dilated lobules.

Conclusion

Extensive fibrosis with lobular type calcifications, typical of cystic hyperplasia.

Histology

Cystic hyperplasia, stromal fibrosis.

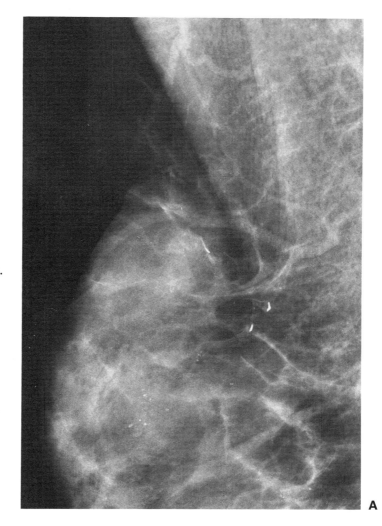

A

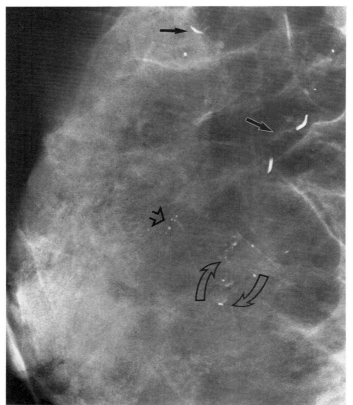

B

114

Age 42, asymptomatic. First screening study.

Physical Examination

No tumor is palpable in the breasts.

Mammography

Fig. 114 A: Right breast, latero-medial projection. Numerous calcifications scattered throughout the breast. No associated tumor.

Fig. 114 B: Right breast, microfocus magnification view, latero-medial projection.

Fig. 114 C: Operative specimen radiograph.

Analysis of the Calcifications

Form: crescent-shaped, teacup-like
Density: uniform, fairly high
Distribution: scattered throughout much of the breast

Conclusion

This is a typical mammographic appearance of the benign-type calcifications seen in cystic hyperplasia.

Histology

Cystic hyperplasia. No epithelial proliferation or atypia.

Comment

The crescent-shaped calcifications (Fig. 114B) appear to resemble a teacup seen from the side. These same calcifications appear circular and smudgy on the specimen radiograph (taken with a vertical x-ray beam) and resemble a teacup seen from above.

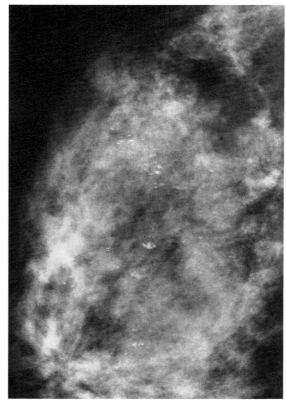

A

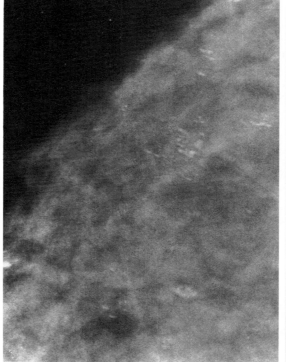

B

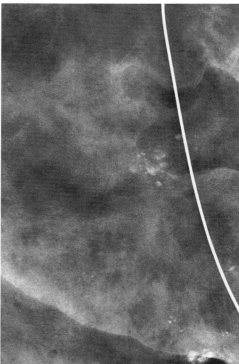

C

115

54-year-old woman, asymptomatic.

Physical Examination

No palpable tumor in the breasts.

Mammography

Fig. 115 A: Microfocus magnification view of the calcifications in the cranio-caudal projection.
Fig. 115 B: Operative specimen radiograph with microfocus magnification.

Analysis of the Calcifications

Form: round, some irregular
Density: difficult to evaluate because of the overlying dense fibrosis; density best evaluated from the operative specimen, where it is fairly uniform
Size: variable
Distribution: within the area of a lobe

Conclusion

Mammographically benign-type calcifications of the lobular type, typical of those seen with cystic hyperplasia.

Histology

Cystic hyperplasia with fibrosis. No epithelial proliferation or atypia.

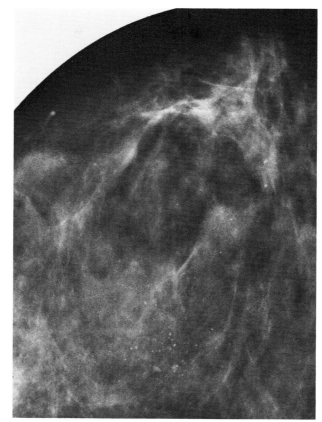

A

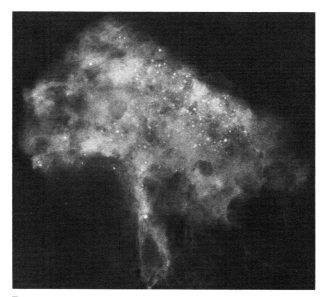

B

116

59-year-old woman, asymptomatic.
First screening study.

Physical Examination

No palpable tumor in the breasts.

Mammography

Fig. 116 A & B: Right breast, medio-lateral oblique and cranio-caudal projections. A large group of calcifications is seen centrally in the breast with no associated tumor (the left breast shows no abnormality).
Fig. 116 C & D: Right breast, micro-focus magnification views, medio-lateral oblique and cranio-caudal projections.

Analysis

Form: round, sharply outlined, lobular type
Density: high, little variation
Distribution: within one lobe
Size: variable, mostly very small

Conclusion

Typical appearance of lobular-type calcifications, mammographically benign. Their distribution and appearance suggest cystic hyperplasia.

Histology

Cystic hyperplasia, fibrosis.

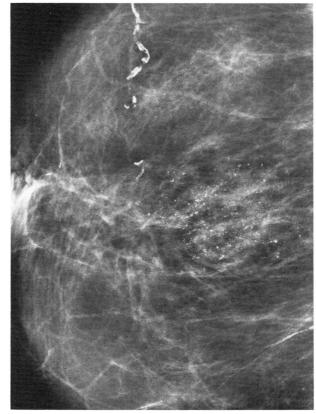

A

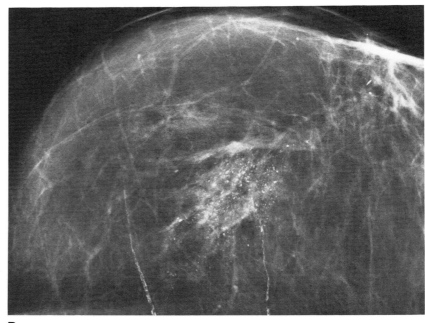

B

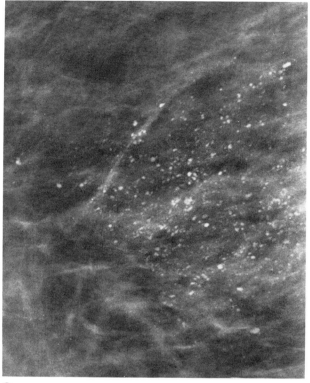

C

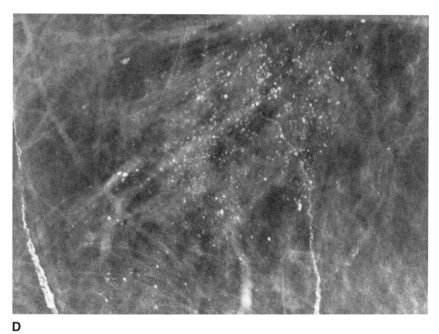

D

117

Asymptomatic, 65-year-old woman. First screening study.

Physical Examination

No palpable tumor in the breasts.

Mammography

Fig. 117: Left breast, medio-lateral oblique projection. Numerous calcifications scattered throughout the breast. No associated tumor.

Analysis

Form: Ring-like, oval, elongated, branching, some needle-like. Sharply outlined, smooth bordered.
Density: High. Nearly all have central lucencies, indicating that they are periductal. The remainder are homogenously calcified.
Distribution: Follow the course of the ducts.

Conclusion

Typical picture of plasma cell mastitis-type calcifications.

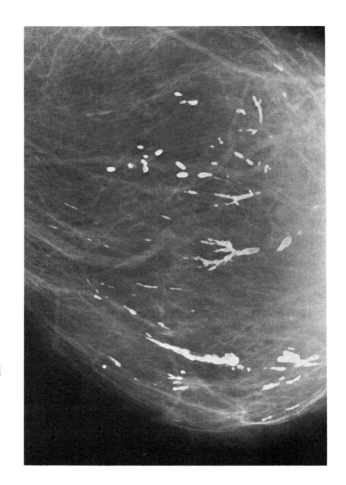

118

Age 64. First screening study. Asymptomatic.

Physical Examination

No palpable tumor in the breasts.

Mammography

Fig. 118 A: Left breast, cranio-caudal projection. In the central portion of the breast there is an approximately 6 × 6 cm area containing numerous calcifications. No associated tumor. Fig. 118 B & C: Microfocus magnification views, cranio-caudal and medio-lateral oblique projections.

Analysis of the Calcifications

Form: mostly elongated, sharply outlined, smooth bordered; some are needle-like
Density: high; some have a lucent central area (periductal calcifications), but most are homogenous in density (solid, intraductal calcifications)
Size: variable
Distribution: some appear to follow the course of a duct

Conclusion

All of the calcifications are mammographically of the benign type. This appearance is of the rarely seen type of plasma cell mastitis, in which most of the calcifications are intraductal.

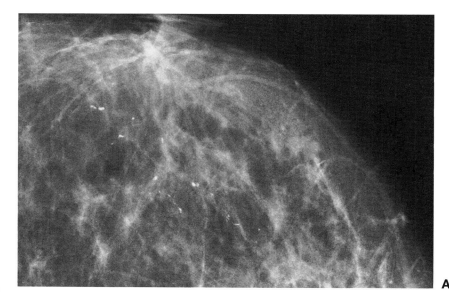

A

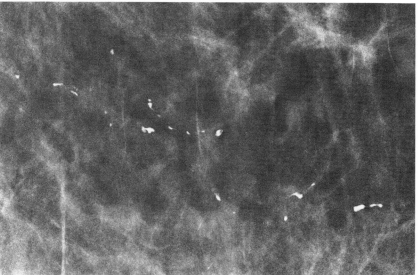

B

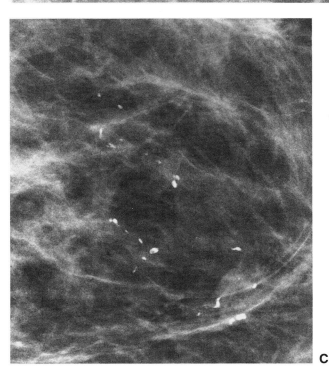

C

119

Age 35, pain in the left breast. No palpable tumor.

Mammography

Fig. 119 A: Right breast, cranio-caudal projection. There are numerous scattered calcifications in the lateral half of the breast. There is extensive fibrosis with no associated tumor.
Fig. 119 B: Microfocus magnification view, cranio-caudal projection.
Fig. 119 C: Operative specimen magnification radiograph.

Analysis of the Calcifications

Form: round, smooth bordered, sharply outlined lobular-type
Density: high, variable (equal sized calcifications are of similar density)
Distribution: in the area of one or two lobes

Conclusion

Typical picture of benign, lobular-type calcifications.

Histology

Sclerosing adenosis.

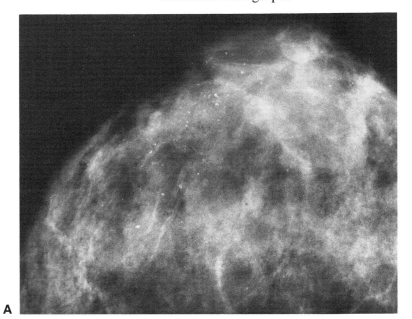

A

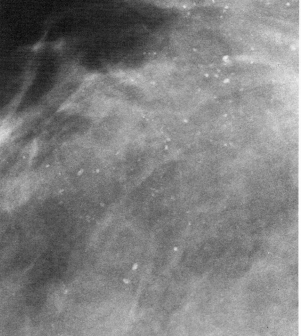

B

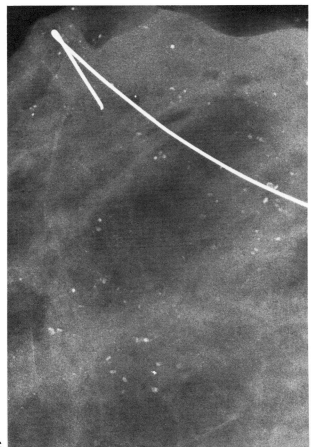

C

120

First screening study, 49-year-old woman.

Physical Examination

No palpable tumor in the breasts.

Mammography

Fig. 120 A: Right breast, medio-lateral oblique projection. Fibrosis throughout the breast. Numerous scattered calcifications of varying size.
Fig. 120 B: Microfocus magnification view, medio-lateral oblique projection.

Analysis of the Calcifications

Form: crescent-shaped, teacup-like; there are also tiny, punctate calcifications
Density: variable, mostly low
Size: variable
Number and distribution: numerous, scattered throughout the breast

Comment

Fibrosis with lobular type calcifications (settling to the dependent portions of dilated lobules) is typical of cystic hyperplasia.

Histology

Cystic hyperplasia. No evidence of malignancy.

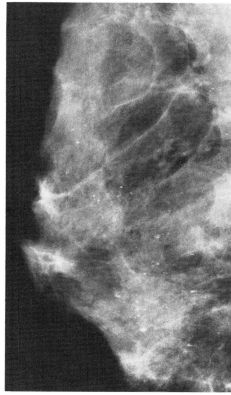

A

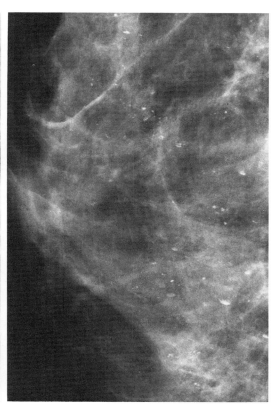

B

121

51-year-old woman, asymptomatic. First screening study.

Physical Examination

No palpable tumor in the breasts.

Mammography

Fig. 121 A & B: Right breast, mediolateral oblique projection, contact (A) and microfocus magnification (B) views.
Fig. 121 C & D: Right breast, craniocaudal projection, contact (C) and microfocus magnification (D) views. Numerous calcifications within a 6 × 6 cm area. No associated tumor. The calcifications are unilateral.

Analysis

Form: round, some needle-like; sharply outlined, smoothly bordered
Density: high, fairly uniform
Size: variable

Conclusion

Typical lobular-type calcifications, mammographically benign. The needle-like calcifications are intraductal but of a benign type because of their homogeneous nature and smooth borders.

Histology

Cystic hyperplasia, sclerosing adenosis, papillomatosis.

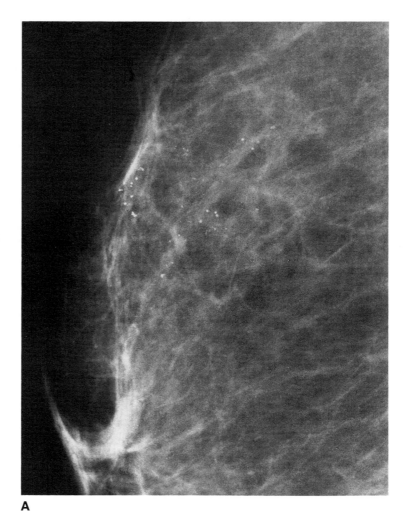

A

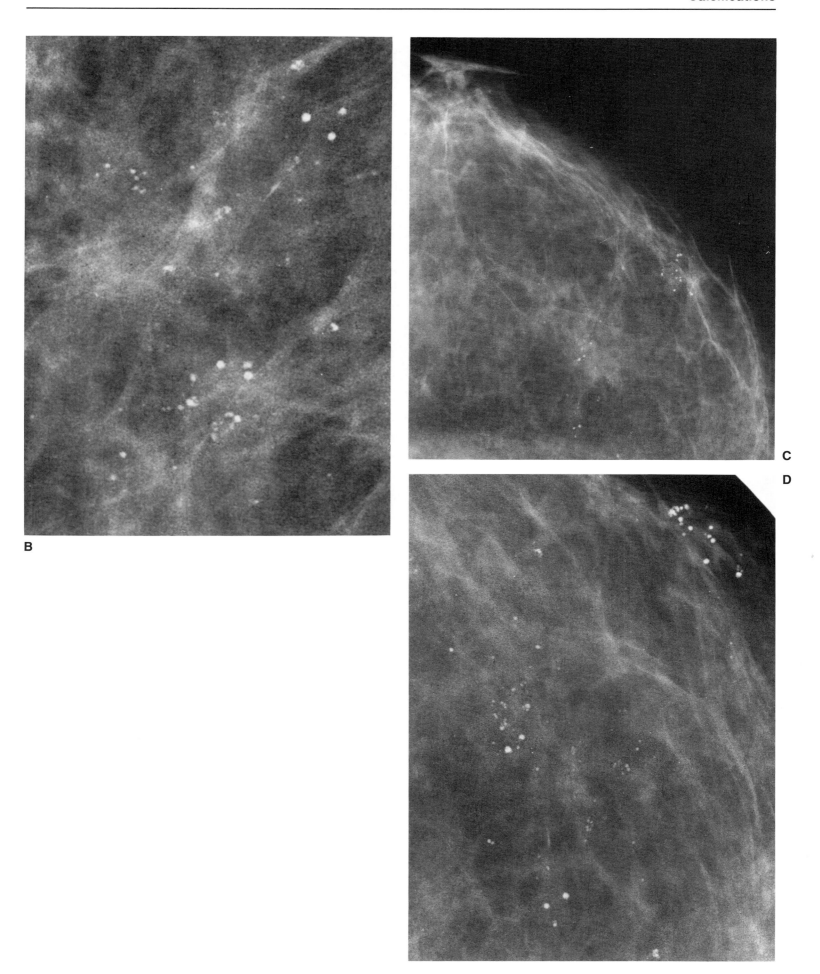

B

C

D

122

First screening examination, 52-year-old asymptomatic woman.

Physical Examination

No palpable tumor in the breasts.

Mammography

Fig. 122 A & B: Right breast, mediolateral oblique projection, contact (A) and microfocus magnification (B) views. There is a 4 × 2 cm area of numerous microcalcifications in the upper half of the breast. No associated tumor.

Analysis of the Calcifications

Form: punctate, smooth contour; typical lobular type calcifications
Density: high, uniform
Size: small, variable
Distribution: localized to an area equal to that of one lobe

Conclusion

Mammographically typical appearance of benign, involutional-type calcifications.

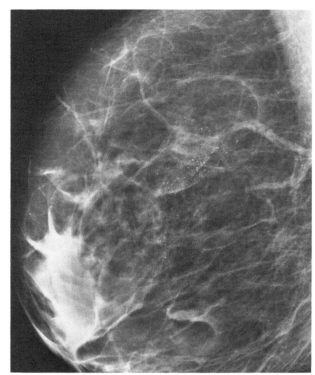

A

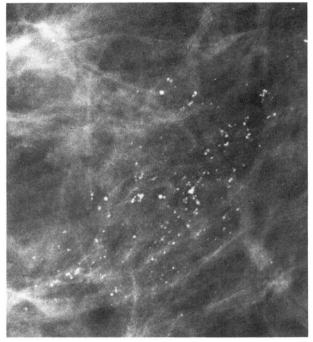

B

123

81-year-old woman, asymptomatic. First screening study.

Physical Examination

No palpable tumor in the breasts.

Mammography

Fig. 123 A: Left breast, medio-lateral oblique projection. Small, centrally located tumor. Calcifications near the nipple, as well as arterial calcifications. Fig. 123 B & C: Enlarged views of the retroareolar region (C) and the centrally located tumor (B), medio-lateral oblique projection.

Analysis of the Tumor

Form: circumscribed, oval
Contour: sharply outlined
Density: radiolucent and radiopaque combined
Size: 9 × 7 mm

Conclusion

This description is typical of an intramammary lymph node.

Analysis of the Calcifications (arrows)

Form: elongated, not fragmented
Density: high, uniform; no hollow centers
Size: length variable, up to 15 mm
Distribution: follow the course of the ducts

Conclusion

Typical appearance of intraductal calcifications resulting from plasma cell mastitis.

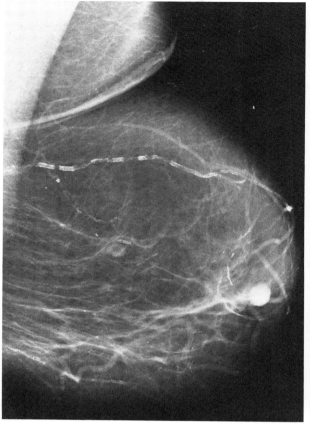

A

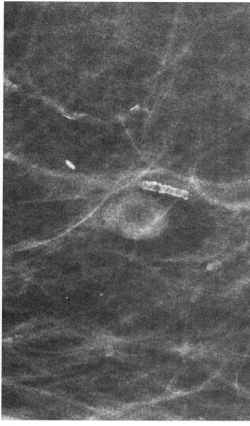

B

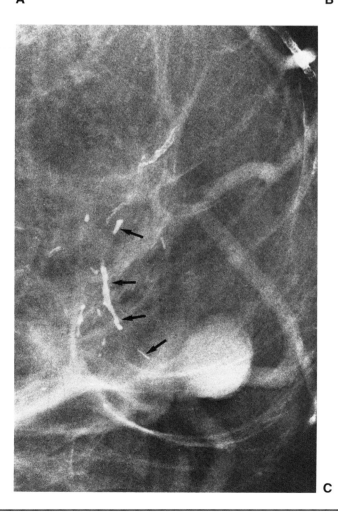

C

124

70-year-old asymptomatic woman, screening study.

Physical Examination

No tumor palpable in the breasts.

Mammography

Fig. 124 A & B: Left breast, medio-lateral oblique projections: numerous scattered calcifications with no associated tumor.
Fig. 124 C: Microfocus magnification view.

Analysis

There are two types of calcifications:
1) The periductal calcifications near the nipple (arrows) are sharply outlined and have high density. These are the plasma cell mastitis-type calcifications.
2) Calcifications seen throughout the mammograms:
   Form: ring-like, oval
   Density: low, lucent center
   Size: same as skin pores
   Number and distribution: numerous, occur within the skin

Comment

Typical picture of calcified sebaceous glands. This unmistakable appearance should never lead to confusion.

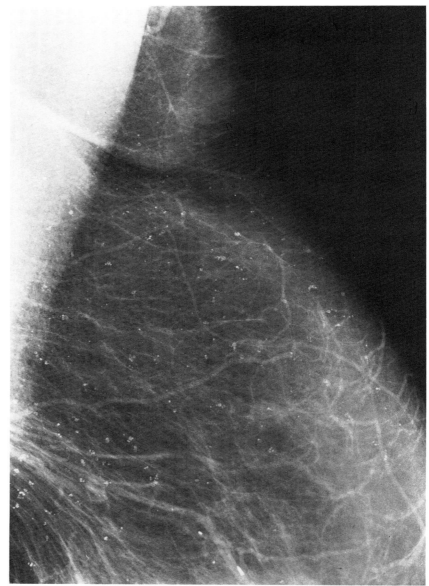

A

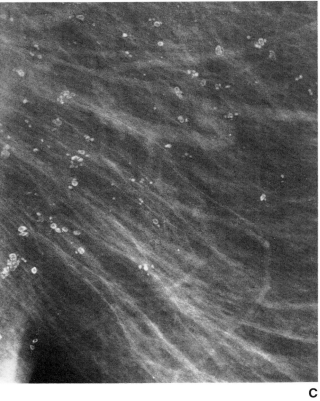

C

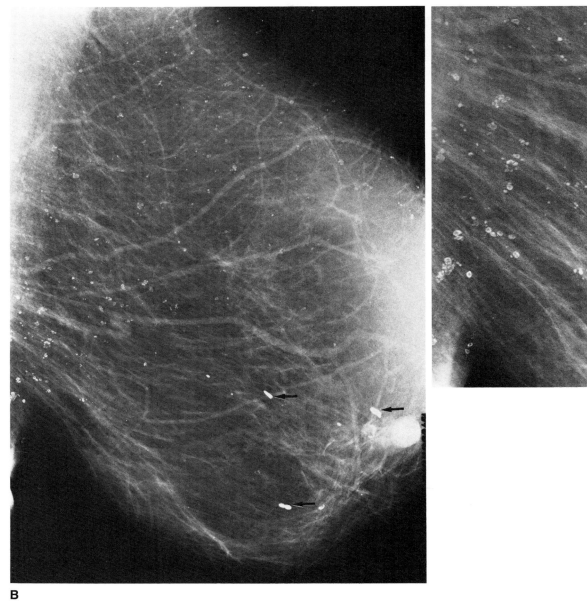

B

125

First screening study, 62-year-old asymptomatic woman.

Physical Examination

No palpable tumor in the breasts.

Mammography

Fig. 125 A & B: Left breast, medio-lateral oblique and cranio-caudal projections. A group of calcifications in the lower half of the breast. No associated tumor.
Fig. 125 C: Microfocus magnification view, cranio-caudal projection.

Analysis of the Calcifications

Form: Irregular, sharply outlined, some elongated.
Density: High, nearly all have central lucencies, indicating that they are periductal. The remainder are uniformly calcified.
Distribution: Localized to a small area, probably following the course of a duct.

Conclusion

Typical mammographic appearance of plasma cell mastitis-type calcifications, localized to a small region.

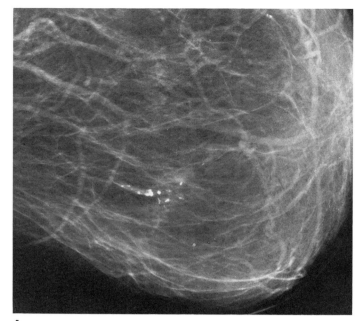

A

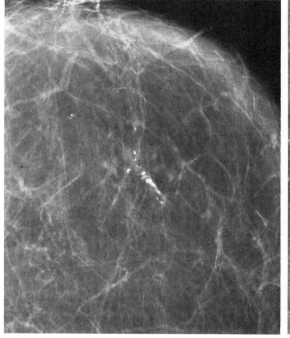

B

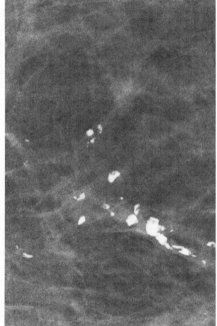

C

126

Age 52, referred for mammography because of cancerophobia.

Physical Examination

No abnormality.

Mammography

Fig. 126 A & B: Left breast, micro-focus magnification views in the medio-lateral oblique and cranio-caudal projections. Scattered calcifications throughout the breast. There were scattered calcifications with extensive fibrosis in the right breast as well.

Analysis of the Calcifications

Form: differ very much from each other, irregular, mostly lobular type
Density: variable
Size: variable
Distribution: scattered throughout the dense parenchyma

Conclusion

It is striking that these lobular-type calcifications are so widely varying in form, size and density. This necessitates thorough histologic examination and future mammographic control. Atypical lobular hyperplasia? Cystic hyperplasia? Lobular cancer in situ?

Histology

Cystic hyperplasia, sclerosing adenosis with intraluminal calcifications. Atypical lobular hyperplasia. No evidence of malignancy.

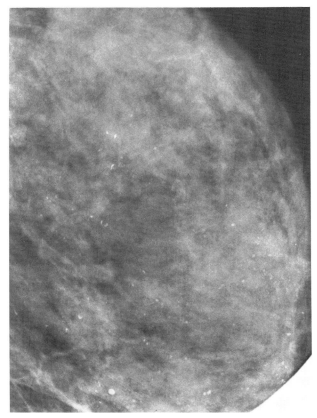

A

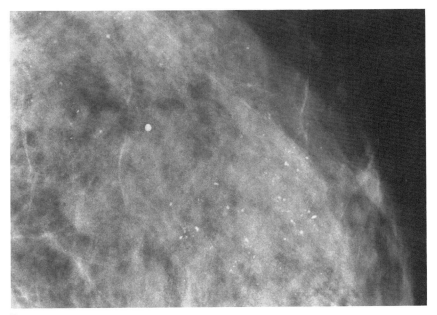

B

127

52-year-old woman, asymptomatic. First Screening examination.

Physical Examination

No palpable tumor in the breasts.

Mammography

Fig. 127 A & B: Left breast, medio-lateral oblique and cranio-caudal projections. Several calcified tumors are seen in the lower outer quadrant of the breast.

Analysis of the Tumors

Form: circumscribed, multilobulated, sharply outlined
Density: low density radiopaque, equal to parenchyma
Size: variable, up to 2 cm
Distribution: appear to lie within the same duct system (within one lobe)

Conclusion

Multiple benign tumors, possibly in one duct and its branches.

Analysis of the Calcifications

Form: irregular, shell-like
Density: variable; larger calcifications very dense, smaller calcifications of variable density
Size: coarse, variable
Distribution: within the tumors

Comment

Benign type calcifications.

Conclusion

Partially calcified multiple benign tumors in the course of one duct and its branches.

Histology

Papillomatosis.

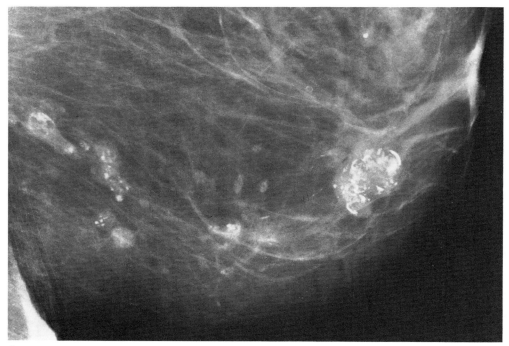

A

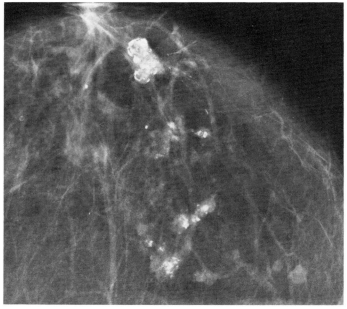

B

128

First screening study, 65-year-old asymptomatic woman.

Physical Examination

No palpable tumor in the breasts.

Mammography

Fig. 128 A: Right breast, cranio-caudal projection: there is a group of calcifications with a surrounding density 5 cm from the nipple.
Fig. 128 B: Microfocus magnification view, cranio-caudal projection.

Analysis of the Tumor

Form: circumscribed, oval
Contour: partly sharply outlined and partly ill-defined, no halo sign
Density: low density radiopaque, equal to that of the parenchyma

Analysis of the Calcifications

Form: highly irregular, but sharply outlined
Density: high, fairly uniform
Size: variable
Distribution: two groups near to each other; one group is not associated with the tumor

Conclusion

Benign type calcifications in a circumscribed tumor with low density.

Histology

Intraductal papillomatosis, calcified. No evidence of malignancy.

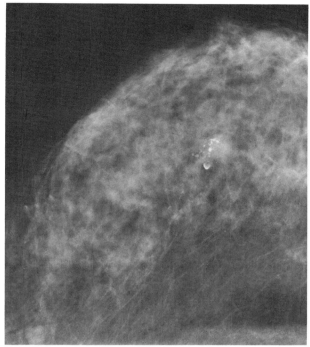

A

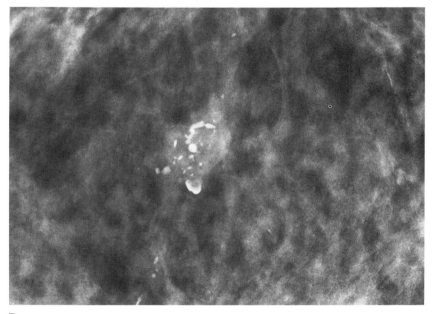

B

129

Fig. 129: Five ring-like calcifications with central lucencies. Sharply outlined, high density, no associated tumor. Typical picture of liponecrosis microcystica calcificans (calcified microhematomas).

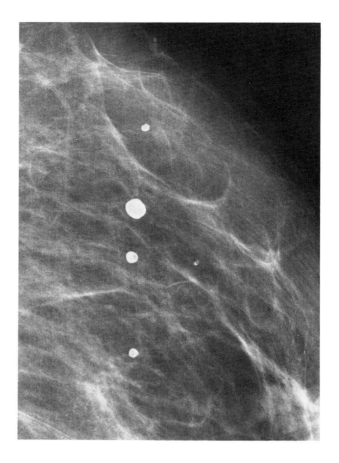

130
131
132

Fig. 130, 131 & 132: Three typical mammographic appearances of totally calcified solitary intraductal papillomas.

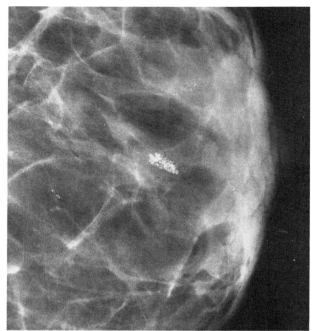

130

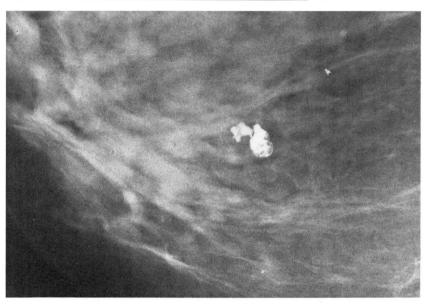

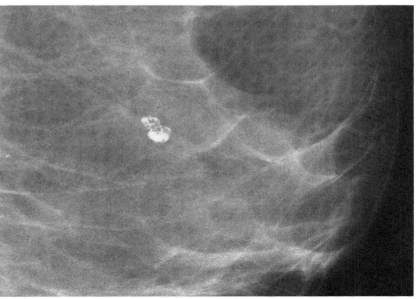

132

133

First screening study, asymptomatic 44-year-old woman.

Physical Examination

No palpable tumor.

Mammography

Fig. 133 A & B: Right and left breasts, medio-lateral oblique projections. Numerous calcifications are seen throughout the breasts.

Analysis

Form: circular
Size: from very small to 3 mm
Density: very dense calcifications with central radiolucencies
Distribution: many if not all of the calcifications lie within the subcutaneous fat

Conclusion

Typical mammographic appearance of liponecrosis microcystica calcificans. These are calcified microhematomas.

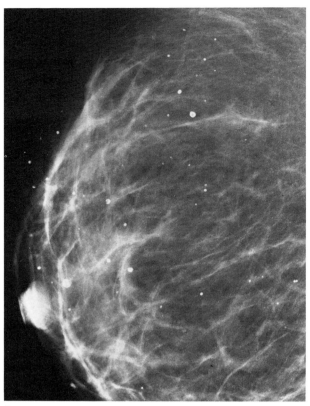

A

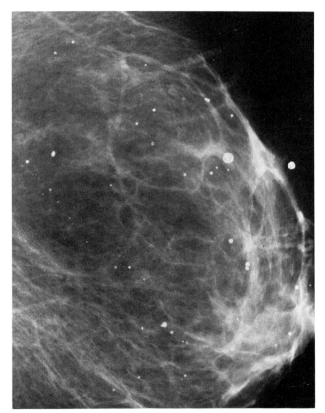

B

134

Breast biopsy 15 years earlier.
Fig. 134: Detailed view in the cranio-caudal projection. There are several large, amorphous calcifications.
Form: irregular, eggshell-like, sharply outlined
Density: high with numerous central radiolucencies
Size: variable, largest 5 × 3 cm

Conclusion

Benign-type calcifications. The history of operation and the central radiolucencies lead to the diagnosis of oil cyst (liponecrosis macrocystica calcificans).

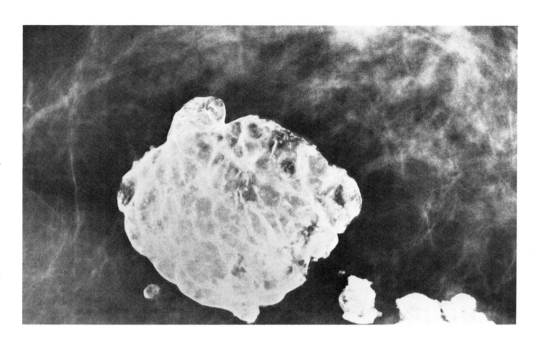

135

58-year-old woman, who underwent plastic surgery to the breast 15 years earlier. First screening examination.

Mammography

Fig. 135: Left breast, cranio-caudal projection. A long subareolar scar is seen adjacent to a calcified lesion.

Analysis

Form: elongated, lobulated, eggshell-like
Size: 3 × 1 cm
Density: high, radiolucent center

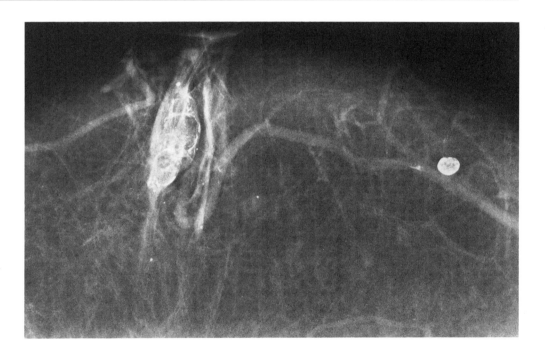

Comment

Cysts, oil cysts and fibroadenomas can all have shell-like calcification, but only the oil cyst has a radiolucent center.

Conclusion

Calcified oil cyst (liponecrosis macrocystica calcificans). The previous operation provides further evidence for this conclusion.
A small calcified oil cyst (liponecrosis microcystica calcificans) is located laterally at the site of the surgical drain.

136

Fig. 136: Cranio-caudal projection. There is a 7 × 6 mm oval shaped circumscribed tumor centrally in the breast (open arrow) with a calcified rim (eggshell-like). This is a partially calcified cyst. There is also a solitary, ring-like calcification (solid arrow) (liponecrosis microcystica calcificans).

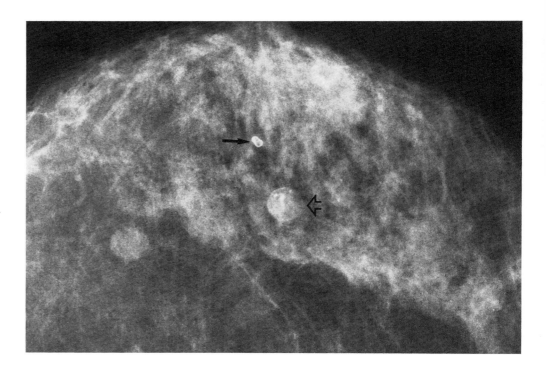

137

78-year-old women, referred for a hard retroareolar tumor, first noted one year earlier.

Mammography

Fig. 137 A & B: Right breast, medio-lateral oblique and cranio-caudal projections. There is a solitary, calcified retroareolar tumor.

Analysis

Form: circumscribed, oval
Contour: sharply outlined, with egg-shell-like calcification
Size: 15 × 20 mm

Comment

An eggshell-like calcified, circum-scribed tumor can be either an oil cyst, a calcified fibroadenoma or a calcified cyst (with or without an intracystic tumor).
1) An oil cyst can be excluded in this case because the contents are not radiolucent.
2) A fibroadenoma has coarse calcifications differing considerably from this lesion (case 138).
3) Cysts calcify in a manner similar to that of this lesion. The thin, faintly calcified shell is the result of bleeding. The bleeding may result from an intracystic growth, especially in lesions located behind the nipple.
Puncture and cytology helps in the final diagnosis.

Cytology

Malignant cells.

Histology

Subareolar papillary carcinoma.

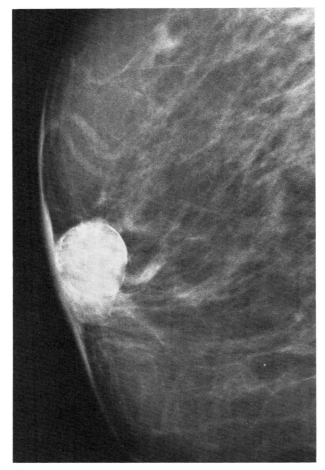

A

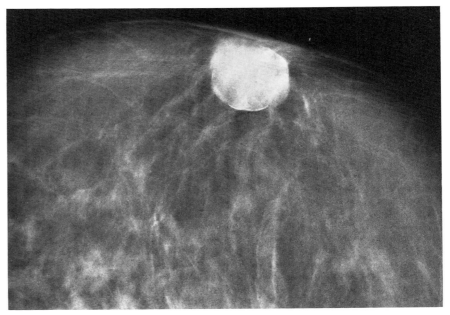

B

138

56-year-old woman, referred to mammography for a calcification seen on the chest X-ray. The patient has been aware of this palpable tumor for many years.

Mammography

Fig. 138 A & B: Left breast, detailed views of the medio-lateral oblique and cranio-caudal projections. A large, calcified tumor is seen immediately behind the nipple.

Analysis of the Tumor

Form: circumscribed, oval, lobulated
Contour: sharply outlined; a halo sign seen along the inferior border of the tumor (arrows)
Density: low density radiopaque, equal to the parenchyma
Size: 3.5 × 3 cm
Location: retroareolar

Comment

On the basis of the above characteristics the tumor is mammographically benign.

Analysis of the Calcifications

Form: eggshell-like, coarse
Density: very high
Location: surround much of the tumor

Conclusion

Benign-type calcifications in a benign tumor, typical of fibroadenoma.

Histology

Calcified fibroadenoma.

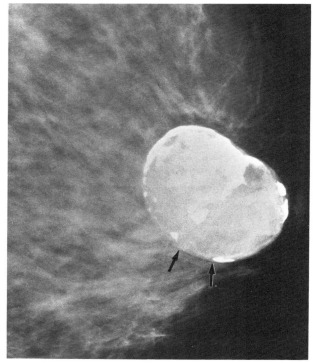

A

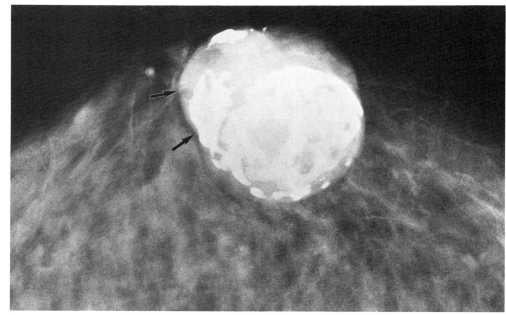

B

139

56-year-old woman, underwent plastic surgery 12 years earlier. The patient has observed gradual nipple retraction on the left side and has noticed a hard retroareolar tumor.

Mammography

Fig. 139 A & B: Left breast, micro-focus magnification views in the medio-lateral oblique and cranio-caudal projections. A large, partially calcified tumor is seen associated with retroareolar fibrosis. The nipple is retracted.

Analysis

Form: circumscribed, lobulated
Contour: partly sharply defined
Density: radiolucent; highly dense eggshell-like calcifications

Conclusion

A radiolucent circumscribed tumor with eggshell-like calcifications and a history of operation leads to the unmistakable diagnosis of oil cyst (liponecrosis macrocystica calcificans).

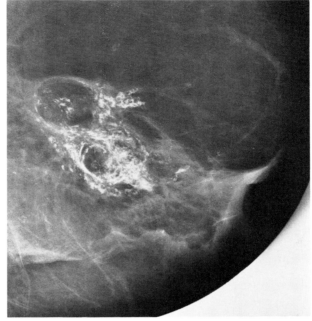

A

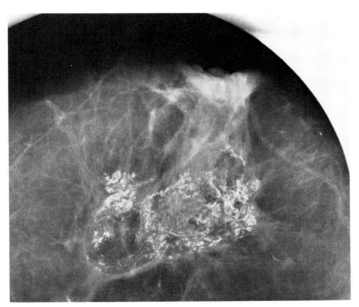

B

140

Fig. 140: Plastic surgery to the breast 15 years earlier. There are several egg-shell-like calcifications, the largest 15 mm. A scar (arrows) extends from the largest calcification to the nipple. The calcified tumors have lucent centers, giving the typical mammographic appearance of liponecrosis macro-cystica calcificans (oil cyst).

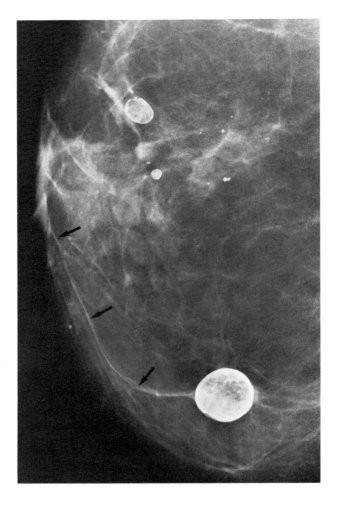

141

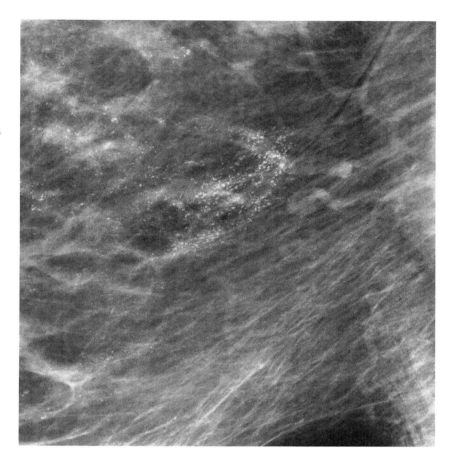

Fig. 141: Detailed view of the medio-lateral oblique projection. Microfocus magnification. Numerous calcifications are seen over an area several cm across. No tumor mass.

Analysis

Form: punctate
Density: high, uniform
Size: extremely small, uniform
Distribution: within one or two lobes

Conclusion

Mammographically benign (involutional-type) calcifications.

142
143
144

Fig. 142, 143 & 144: Three examples of hyalinized fibroadenomas. The calcifications are coarse, amorphous, sharply outlined and of extremely high density. The calcifications are situated within a mammographically benign tumor.

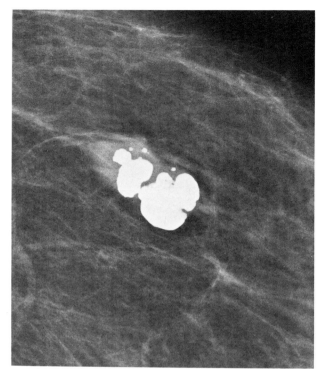

142

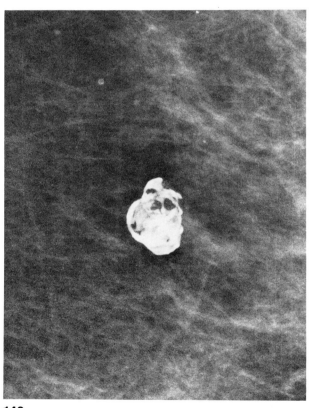

143

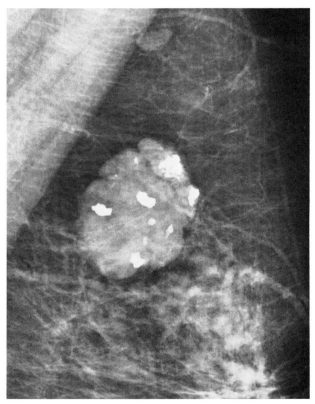

144

145– 149

Fig. 145, 146, 147, 148 & 149: In contrast to the coarse calcifications associated with the myxoid degeneration of a fibroadenoma, these calcifications, located superficially within a fibroadenoma, may lead to diagnostic difficulties. When they are small and numerous they may easily be confused with malignant-type calcifications (granular type).

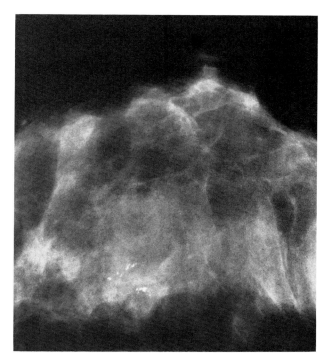

145 A

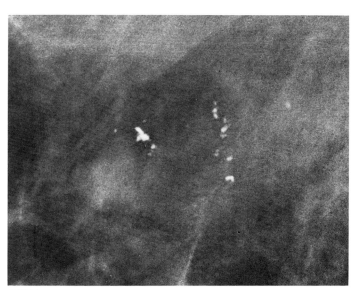

145 B

Fig. 146–149 ▷

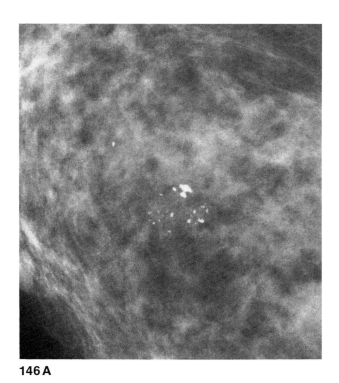

146 A

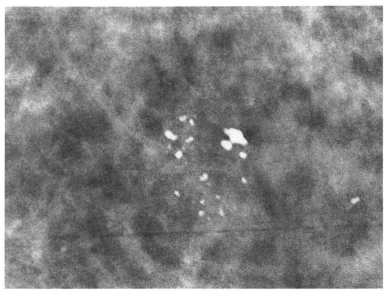

146 B

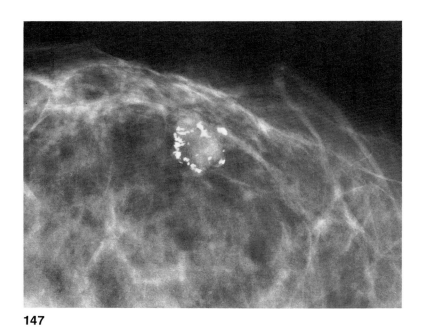

147

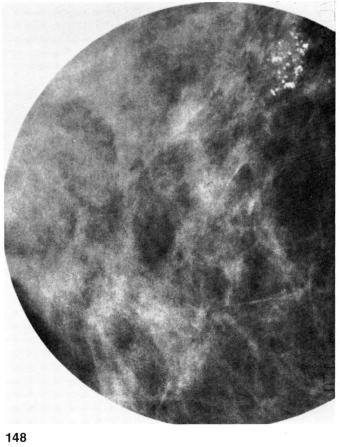

148

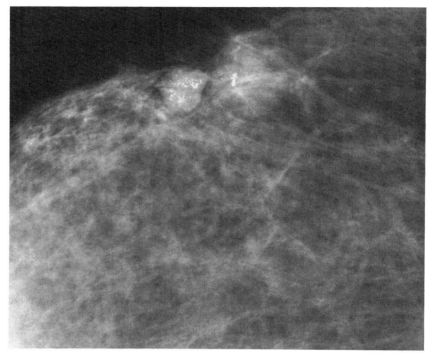

149 A

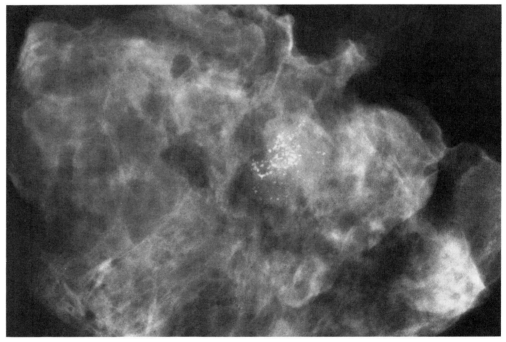

149 B

150

This 63-year-old woman noted a lump in her right breast, below the areola, six month earlier.

Physical Examination

Freely moveable 1 cm tumor, clinically benign.

Mammography

Fig. 150 A & B: Coned-down compression views of the tumor, which is associated with calcifications.

Analysis of the Tumors

Form: circumscribed, oval, slightly lobular
Contour: unsharp, no halo sign; there is a small comet tail (arrows, Fig. 150 A)
Density: low density radiopaque
Size: 10 × 10 mm

Analysis of the Calcifications

Form: coarse, irregular
Density: high
Distribution: eggshell-like (partially)

Conclusion

the calcifications are of the benign type (reminiscent of a partially calcified fibroadenoma). The tumor, although of low density, is not sharply outlined, the halo sign is missing and there is a comet tail. This necessitates biopsy.

Histology

Carcinoma in an old, hyalinized fibroadenoma.

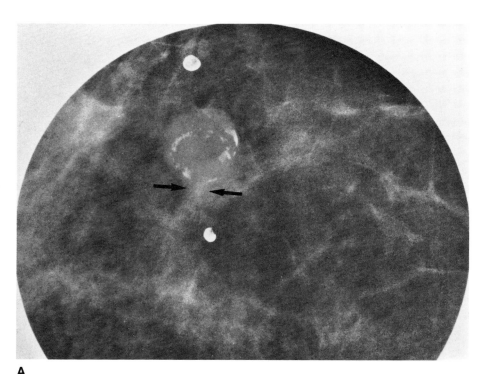

A

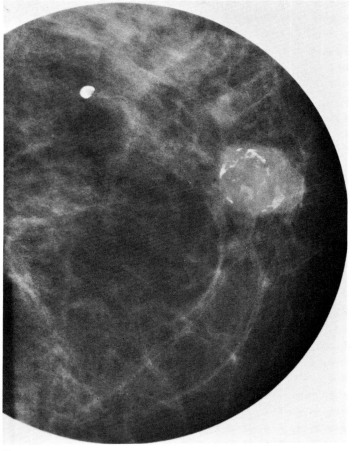

B

151

First screening examination. 61-year-old woman.

Physical Examination

Hard, freely movable tumor in the upper inner quadrant of the right breast. The tumor had been present for 20 years; the overlying skin is bluish.

Mammography

Fig. 151 A: Right breast, craniocaudal projection. A calcified tumor is seen in the upper inner quadrant.
Fig. 151 B & C: Enlarged coned-down compression views before and after puncture.

Analysis of the Tumor

Form: circumscribed, lobulated
Contour: sharply outlined, halo sign seen
Density: low density radiopaque, parenchymal structures can be seen superimposed
Size: large, 4 × 3 cm

Conclusion

Mammographically benign tumor.

Analysis of the Calcifications

Form: highly irregular, bizarre
Density: high
Size: coarse, variable
Location: inside the tumor

Conclusion

The extremely high density and coarseness indicate a benign character.

Puncture

Several ml dark blood aspirated. Note the defect at the site of puncture (arrows).

Cytology

Blood, no epithelial elements.

Histology

Calcified hemangioma. No evidence of malignancy.

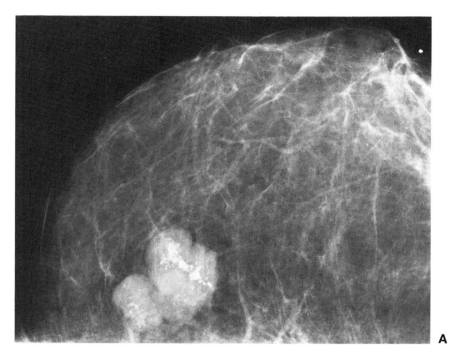

A

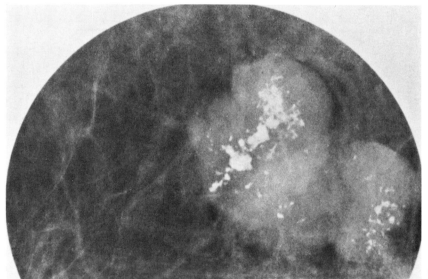

B

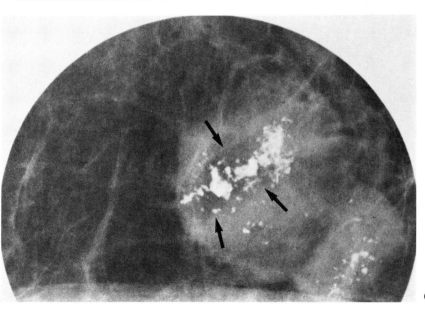

C

152

Fig. 152 A & B: Calcified wart in the medio-lateral and cranio-caudal projections. The calcifications are deceptive.

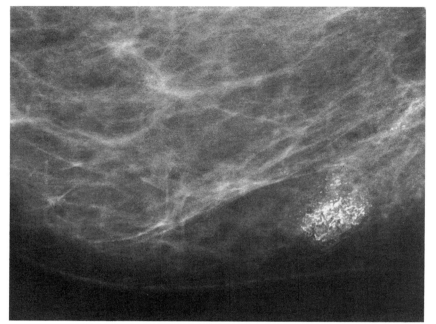

A

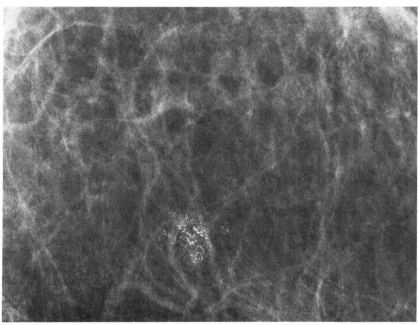

B

VII. Thickened Skin Syndrome of the Breast

This is a syndrome produced by lymphedema usually secondary to obstruction of the axillary lymphatics (Fig. XXI).

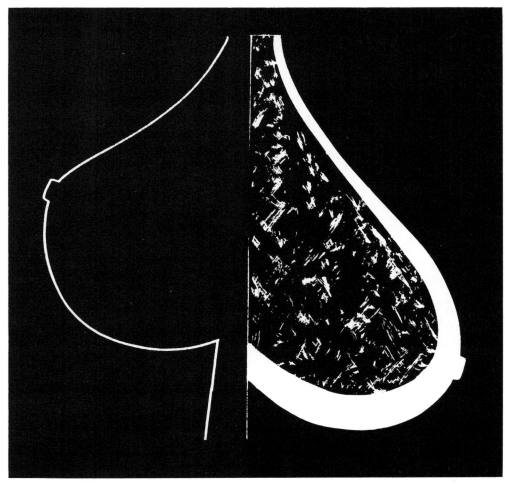

Fig. XXI: Thickened skin syndrome: Thickened skin over much or all of the breast, associated with increased density and a reticular pattern.

Physical Examination

a) The affected breast is larger and heavier due to increased fluid content.
b) There is obvious *peau d'orange*.
c) Enlarged axillary lymph nodes are frequently palpable.
d) The skin is inflamed in the so-called inflammatory carcinoma, in acute mastitis and frequently in abscesses.

Mammographic Appearance

a) The skin is obviously thickened, usually many times normal thickness. This occurs initially and to the greatest extent in the lower, dependent portion of the breast.
b) The overall density of the breast is increased due to the high fluid content. In comparison to the other breast there is a coarse reticular pattern on the mammogram.

Lymphedema May be Caused by the Following:

a) Axillary lymphatic obstruction blocking lymphatic drainage of the breast. This may be secondary to:
   1) Breast carcinoma metastases. In many cases an aggressive carcinoma may spread throughout the breast and axilla (case 153). A carcinoma may also be located high in the axillary tail and metastasize directly to the axillary lymph nodes.
   2) Primary malignant lymphatic diseases (lymphomas, etc.).
   3) Advanced gynecological malignancies (ovarian, uterine) which may rarely block primary lymphatic drainage in the lesser pelvis (37). The lymph flow then passes through the thoraco-epigastric collaterals, overloading the axillary and supraclavicular lymphatic drainage (case 154).
   4) Advanced bronchial or esophageal carcinoma may cause blockage of the mediastinal lymph drainage, also resulting in the thickened skin syndrome of the breast(s).
b) Lymphatic spread of breast carcinoma cells from mastectomy side towards the opposite breast. This spread blocks intradermal and intramammary lymph channels in the remaining breast.
c) Inflammation, particularly large retromammillary abscesses that may produce skin thickening over the areola and the lower part of the breast. An important differentiating factor is that the axillary portion of the breast does not then show the reticular pattern on the mammogram (cases 38, 42).
d) Right heart failure, chonic renal failure, anasarca. This may be restricted to one breast in a bedridden patient lying on one side.

153

62-year-old woman noted increase in size of the right breast over the past six months.

Physical Examination

The right breast is erythematous, heavy and remarkably larger than the left. There is *peau d'orange* and an enlarged axillary lymph node is palpable. The left breast is normal.

Mammography

Fig. 153: Right breast, cranio-caudal projection. Extreme skin thickening over the entire breast. Extensive, prominent reticular pattern. No localized tumor. No associated calcifications.

Conclusion

An extensive reticular pattern reflects lymphedema resulting from obstruction of the axillary lymphatics. Massive lymphedema usually results from axillary lymphatic obstruction by malignant disease. In the absence of a tumor mass one should suspect a diffusely infiltrating malignant breast tumor.

Histology

Diffusely infiltrating breast carcinoma. Metastases to the axillary lymph nodes.

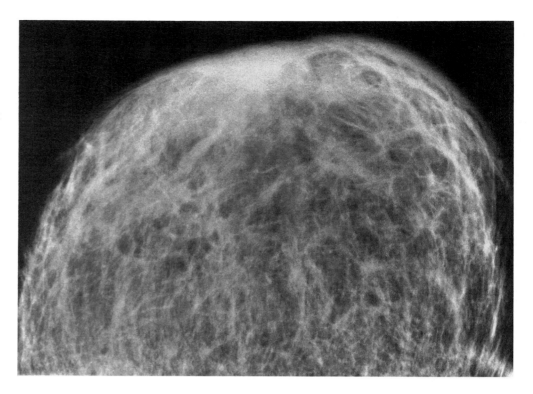

154

72-year-old woman, metastatic ovarian carcinoma operated and irradiated four months earlier.

Physical Examination

The patient now has enlarged, hard axillary and supraclavicular lymph nodes. Both breasts are heavy and erythematous with *peau d'orange*.

Mammography

Fig. 154 A: Left breast, medio-lateral oblique projection.
Fig. 154 B: Right breast, cranio-caudal projection.
Extreme bilateral skin thickening, increased radiopacity and extensive reticular pattern throughout both breasts. No localized tumor, no associated calcifications.

Conclusion

The history is crucial in this case. Advanced gynecological malignancies (uterine and ovarian) as in this case may block the lymphatic drainage in the lesser pelvis. The lymph flow then passes through the thoracoepigastric collaterals, overloading the axillary and supraclavicular lymphatics. This leads to lymphatic stasis in the breasts which accounts for the above-described clinical and mammographic picture.

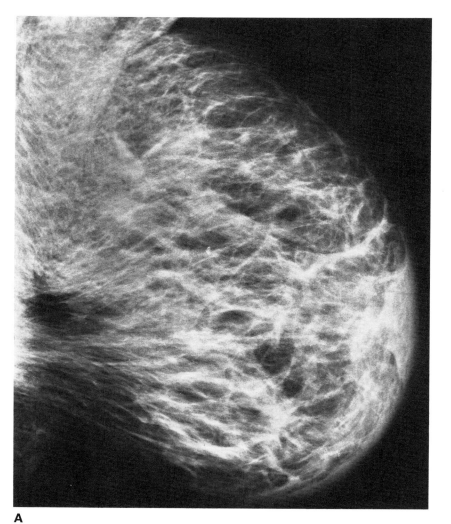

A

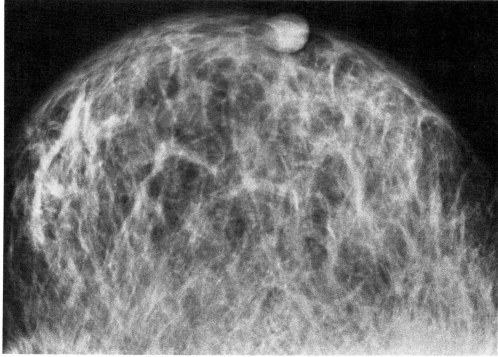

B

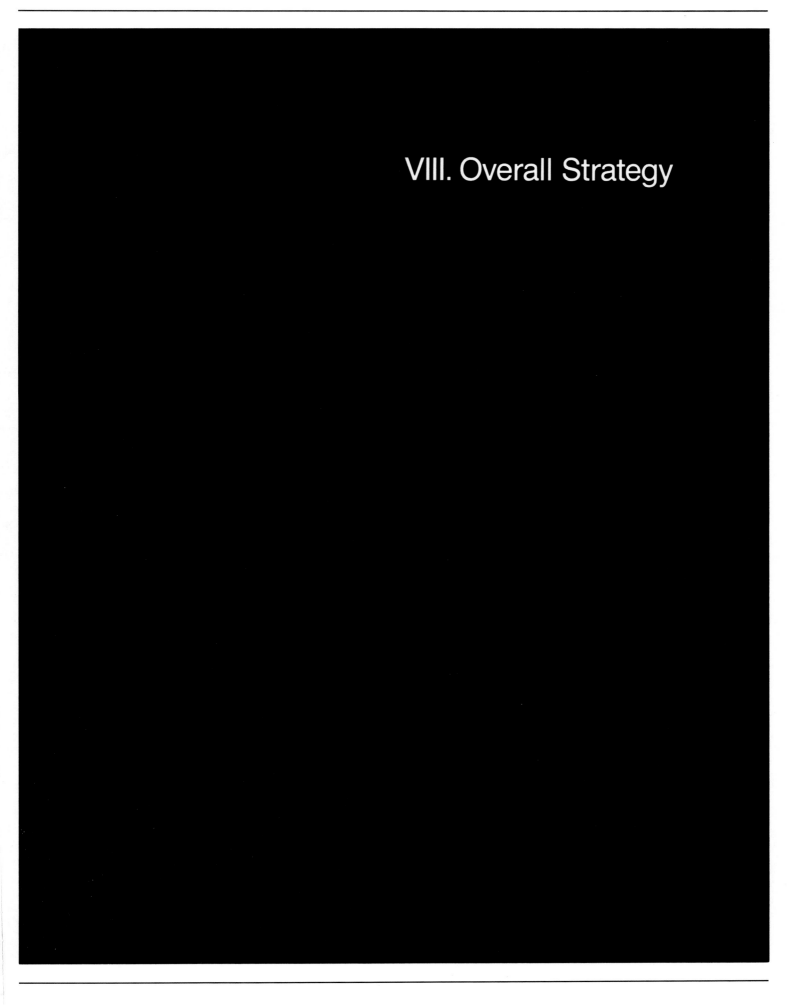

VIII. Overall Strategy

Perception of pathological lesions in the breast can be difficult, especially of stellate tumors. Superior picture quality, optimal viewing conditions and a systematic viewing technique are prerequisite to the perception of breast abnormalities.

Analysis of the perceived lesion should be carefully performed as outlined. The strategy differs according to the type of the tumor:

a) *Circumscribed tumors:* Usually no perception problem. Careful analysis is required because surgical biopsy is often unnecessary. The most striking example of this is the cyst, of which at least 95% can be cured by pneumocystography alone (24, 39, 45).

b) *Stellate Lesions:* Most breast carcinomas present as stellate tumors. Finding them in the early stage when they are small (< 10 mm) may cause considerable perception problems. Once perceived, definitive diagnosis can be made only by histology, although radiological differential diagnosis can be highly accurate.

c) Most *calcifications* in the breast represent benign processes. Since *only 20%* of consecutively biopsied clusters of calcifications represent malignant disease (9, 12), detailed mammographic analysis of the calcifications may help to avoid many unnecessary surgical biopsies.

d) The *thickened skin syndrome* presents with a striking clinical and mammographic appearance. The underlying cause of this syndrome can be determined through careful analysis of the clinical and mammographic picture.

References

1 Ahmed, A.: Calcifications in human breast carcinomas: ultrastructural observations. J Pathol 117:247−251, 1975

2 Ahmed, A.: Atlas of the ultrastructure of human breast diseases. Churchill Livingstone, Edinburgh & New York 1978

3 Andersson, I.: Mammographic screening for breast carcinoma. Dissertation. Malmö 1980

4 Azzopardi, J. G.: Problems in breast pathology. Saunders, Philadelphia 1980

5 Baclesse, F., A. Willemin: Atlas of mammography. Literaire des Facultés, Paris 1967

6 Barth, V.: Atlas of diseases of the breast. Thieme, Stuttgart 1979

7 Bjurstam, N. G.: Radiography of the female breast and axilla. Acta Radiol. Supl. 357. Stockholm 1978

8 Black, J. W., B. Young: A radiological and pathological study of the incidence of calcification in diseases of the breast and neoplasms of other tissues. B J Radiol 38:596, 1965

9 Citoler, P.: Microcalcifications of the breast. In: Grundmann, E., ed.: Early diagnosis of breast cancer. G. Fischer, New York 1978, pp 113−118

10 Dossett, J. A.: In: Risk factors in breast cancer. New aspects of breast cancer (B. A. Stoll, ed.). Heinemann, London 1976, Vol. 2, pp 54−66

11 Egan, R. L.: Mammography, Thomas, Springfield, Ill. 1964

12 Egan, R. L., M. B. Mc Sweeney, C. W. Sewell: Intramammary calcifications without an associated mass in benign and malignant disease. Radiology 137:1, 1980

13 Evans, K. T., I. H. Gravelle: Mammography, thermography and ultrasonography in breast diseases. Butterworths, London 1973

14 Fenoglio, C., R. Lattes: Sclerosing papillary proliferation in the female breast. A benign lesion often mistaken for carcinoma. Cancer (Philad.) 33:691, 1974

15 Fisher, E. R., A. S. Palekar, N. Kotwol, N. Lipana: A nonencapsulated sclerosing lesion of the breast. Am J Clin Pathol 71:240, 1979

16 Frank, H. A., F. M. Hall, M. L. Steer: Preoperative localisation of non-palpable breast lesions demonstrated by mammography. New Engl J Med 295:259, 1976

17 Frischbier, H. J., U. Lohbeck: Frühdiagnostik des Mammakarzinoms. Thieme, Stuttgart 1977

18 Gad, A.: Personal communication

19 Gershon-Cohen, J.: Atlas of mammography. Springer, Berlin 1970

20 Goes, J. S., Jr., J. C. G. S. Goes: Diagnostico Radiologico das doeucasda mama. Livraria Editora, 1979

21 Grassigli, A., A. Grosso, U. Luchini: Infiltrative sclerosing adenosis of the breast. A benign lesion often mistaken for carcinoma. Surgery in Italy Vol. 7, No. 4, 1977

22 Gros, Ch. M.: Les maladies du sein. Masson, Paris 1963

23 Haagensen, C. D., N. Lane, R. Lattes: Neoplastic proliferations of the mammary lobules. Surg Clin Noth Amer 52:497, 1972

24 Hoeffken, W., M. Lányi: Mammography. Thieme, Stuttgart 1977

25 Hoeffken, W., M. Lányi: Erkrankungen der Brustdrüse. In: Schinz: Lehrbuch der Röntgendiagnostik, Band II, Teil 2. Thieme, Stuttgart 1981, pp 969−1041

26 Ingleby, H., J. Gershon-Cohen: Comparative anatomy, pathology and roentgenology of the breast. University of Pennsylvania Press, Philadelphia 1960

27 Lányi, M., P. Citoler: Differentialdiagnose der Mikroverkalkungen: Die kleincystische (blunt duct) Adenose. Fortschr Röntgenstr 134:225, 1981

28 Leborgne, R. A.: Esteatonecrosis quistica calcificata de la mama. Torax 16:172, 1967

29 Leborgne, R. A.: Diagnosis of tumors of the breast by simple roentgenography: calcifications in carcinomas. AJR 65:1, 1951

30 Leborgne, R. A.: The breast in roentgen diagnosis. Impresora Uruguaya, Montevideo 1953

31 Levitan, L. H., D. M. Witten, E. G. Harrison: Calcification in breast disease. Mammographic-pathologic correlation. AJR 92:29, 1964

32 Linell, F., O. Ljungberg, I. Andersson: Breast carcinoma. Aspects of early stages, progression and related problems. Munksgaard, Copenhagen 1980

33 Lundgren, B.: Malignant features of breast tumors at radiography. Acta Radiol Diagn 19:623, 1978

34 Luzzatti, G., B. Salvadori, E. Tavani: Xeromammography. Excerpta Medica, Amsterdam 1979

35 Martin, J. E.: Breast calcifications − benign or malignant? In: Diagnostic Radiology − 1977. Univ. of Calif. at San Francisco 1978

36 Millis, R., R. Davis, A. J. Stacey: The detection and significance of calcifications in the breast: a radiological and pathological study. Br J Radiol 49:12, 1976

37 Martin, J. E., M. Moskowitz, J. R. Milbrath: Breast cancer missed by mammography. AJR 132:737, 1979

38 Molnár, Z., G. Keller: Kollaterale Lymphbahnen der Thoraxwand bei tumoröser Blockade im kleinen Becken. Fortschr Röntgenstr 111:854, 1969

39 Muller, J. W. Th.: Management of benign looking breast lesions. Diagnostic and therapeutic puncture of mammary cysts. In: International symposium on intervention radiology. Lisbon 1979

40 Péntek, Z., J. Balogh, B. Bakó, et al: Maligne Papillomatose in einer riesigen Brustzyste. Fortschr Röntgenstr 120: 756, 1974

41 Rickert, R. R., L. Kalisher, R. V. P. Hutter: Indurative mastopathy: a benign sclerosing lesion of breast with elastosis which may simulate carcinoma. Cancer 47:561, 1981

42 Sickles, E. A.: Microfocal spot magnification mammography using xeroradiographic and screen-film recording systems. Radiology 131:599, 1979

43 Tabár, L., P. B. Dean: Interventional procedures in the investigation of lesions of the breast. Radiol Clin North Am 17:607, 1979

44 Tabár, L., Z. Péntek: Pneumocystography of benign and malignant intracystic growth of the female breast. Acta Radiol Diagn 17:829, 1976

45 Tabár, L., Z. Péntek, P. B. Dean: The diagnostic and therapeutic value of breast cyst puncture and pneumocystography. Radiology 141:659, 1981

46 Tabár, L.: Detection of early breast cancers with complex roentgenologic methods (In Hungarian). Dissertation. Univ of Pécs, Hungary 1978

47 Tremblay, G., R. H. Buell, R. A. Seemayer: Elastosis in benign sclerosing ductal proliferation of the female breast. Amer J Surg Pathology 1:155, 1977

48 Wellings, S. R., H. M. Jensen, R. G. Marcum: An atlas of subgross pathology of the human breast with special reference to possible precancerous lesions. J Natl Cancer Inst 55:231, 1975

49 Wellings, S. R., J. N. Wolfe: Correlative studies of the histological and radiographic appearance of the breast parenchyma. Radiology 129:299, 1978

50 Wellings, S. R.: Development of human breast cancer. Advances in cancer research, Vol. 31, pp 287−314, 1980

51 Willemin, A.: Mammographic appearances. Karger, Basel 1972

52 Wolfe, J. N.: Mammography. Thomas, Springfield, Ill. 1967

53 Sickles, E. A., J. S. Abele: Milk of calcium within tiny benign breast cysts. Radiology 141:655, 1981

54 Sickles, E. A., D. L. Klein, W. H. Goodson, III, T. K. Hunt: Mammography after needle aspiration of palpable breast masses. Am J Surg 145:395, 1983

55 Tabár, L., P. B. Dean, Z. Péntek: Galactography: the diagnostic procedure of choice for nipple discharge. Radiology 149:31, 1983

Index

A

abscess 64, 70
– aspiration 64, 70
adenosis *2, 3*, 170
– sclerosing 154, 170, 182, 191
atheroma (sebaceous cyst) 18, 19, 44, 54

B

breast, anatomy 2
– – lobe 2
– – lobule *2*, 170, 171
– – terminal ductal lobular unit (TDLU) 2
– – ducts 2, 138
– – ductules 2, 138

C

calcifications 138, 139, 170–173, 218
– analysis 138–210
– arterial 173
– atypical lobular hyperplasia 171, 191
– casting type *138, 139*, 143–148, 153, 154, 157–160, 162–165, 168, 169
– comedo carcinoma 140, 144, 146, 160, 165, 168
– crescent shaped 142
– cyst 172, 198
– cystic hyperplasia 170, 171, 174–178, 183, 184, 191
– ductal type 138–169
– eggshell like *172*, 197–202, 208
– fibroadenoma 169, 172, 173, 200, 204–208
– granular type 138–143, 146, 150, 152–154, 164, 165, 168
– hemangioma 45, 209
– involutional type *171, 172*, 186, 203
– liponecrosis macrocystica calcificans 24, 172, 184, 197, 201
– – microcystica calcificans 24, 152, 172, 194, 196–198
– lobular type 154, 170–172, 174–178, 182–184, 191
– miscellaneous 172, 173
– oil cyst 4, *172*, 197, 201, 202
– papilloma 173, 195
– papillomatosis 173, 192, 193
– plasma cell mastitis type 104, 159, 172, 180, 181, 187, 190
– punctate 138, 175, 186, 203
– sclerosing adenosis 154, 170, 182, 191
– sebaceous gland 172, 188, 189
– teacup shaped 170, 175, 176, 183
– warts 210
carcinoma 18, 19, 51, 56, 88, 89, 138
– comedo infiltrating 128, 140, 146
– – noninfiltrating 144, 160, 168
– diffusely infiltrating 214
– ductal infiltrating 143, 145, 148, 157, 166, 169
– – with minimal invasion 150, 152, 163, 165
– – noninvasive 60, 142, 154, 156, 158, 159, 164
– – within a fibroadenoma 162, 173, 208
– lobular in situ 170
– medullary 66
– mucinous 18, 19, 50, 55, 74
– Paget's disease 164
– papillary 18, 19, 69, 199
– scirrhous 88–92, 94, 95, 110, 112, 114, 116, 118, 120, 122, 124, 126, 127, 136
– tubular 102
circumscribed lesions, analysis 18–86
– strategy 218
comet tail sign 56, 136, 208
cyst 2, 3, 18, 19
– aspiration 20, 37, 38, 42, 67, 84, 86
– calcified 172, 198
– differential diagnosis 18, 19, 199
– intracystic tumor 18, 66, 199
– oil cyst 18, 19, 23, 172, 197, 201, 202
– pneumocystography 20, 37, 38, 42, 66, 84, 86
– sebaceous cyst (atheroma) 18, 19, 44, 54
cystic hyperplasia 2, 3, 170, 171, 174–178, 183, 184, 191
cystosarcoma phylloides 18, 19, 63
– – calcified 47

E

epitheliosis 2

F

fibro-adeno-lipoma 18, 19, 25
– differential diagnosis 28
fibroadenoma 18, 19, 32–34, 52, 59, 80–82, 84
– calcified 169, 172, 173, 200, 204–208
– carcinoma within a fibroadenoma 162, 173, 208
– differential diagnosis 18, 19, 172, 199
fine needle puncture 20, 37, 38, 42, 67, 77, 84, 86, 209
foreign body granuloma 109

G

galactocele 18, 19, 26, 27
– differential diagnosis 28
galactography 48
giant fibroadenoma 18, 19, 43

H

halo sign 18, 36, 37, 43, 47, 80, 81, 83, 84, 86
hemangioma 45, 209
hematoma 18, 19, 30, 31, 77
– differential diagnosis 28

I

intramammary lymph node 18, 19, 28, 29, 187
– differential diagnosis 28, 78

L

lipoma 18, 19, 21, 22
liponecrosis macrocystica calcificans 24, *172*, 197, 201, 202
– microcystica calcificans 24, 152, *172*, 194, 196–198
localization, preoperative 56–58
lymph node enlargement, axilla, rheumatoid arthritis 72
– – leukaemia 76
lymphedema 212, 213
lymphoma, metastatic to the breast 62

M

melanoma, metastatic to the breast 68
metastases to the breast, lymphoma 62
– – melanoma 68

P

Paget's disease 164
papilloma, calcified 173, 195
papillomatosis 48
– calcified 173, 192, 193
– juvenile 79
parenchymal retraction 10–12, 14, 112, 124, 127, 128
peau d'orange 70, 213–215
plasma cell mastitis type calcifications *172*
– intraductal 104, 159, 172, 181, 187
– periductal 172, 180, 181, 190
pneumocystography 20, 37, 38, 42, 66, 84, 86

R

reticular pattern on mammograms 212–215

S

sclerosing duct hyperplasia *89, 90*, 96, 98–100, 104, 129, 130

– – – calcified 106
– – – combined with carcinoma 133
– – – differential diagnosis 97
sebaceous cyst 18, 19, 44, 54
skin, retraction 95, 109, 134
– thickening 95, 109, 212–214
stellate lesions, analysis 88–136
– – strategy 218

T

tent sign *12*, 13, 14, 112, 128
thickened skin syndrome *212*, *213*, 214, 215,
   218
traumatic fat necrosis *90*, 105, 108, 134, 172

V

viewing of mammograms 6–14

W

warts 46
– calcified 210